Horse
Business Management
Managing a Successful Yard

Second Edition

Jeremy Houghton Brown
and
Vincent Powell-Smith

**Blackwell
Science**

© Jeremy Houghton Brown
and Ingramlight Properties Ltd 1989, 1995

Blackwell Science Ltd
Editorial Offices:
Osney Mead, Oxford OX2 0EL
25 John Street, London WC1N 2BL
23 Ainslie Place, Edinburgh EH3 6AJ
238 Main Street, Cambridge
  Massachusetts, 02142, USA
54 University Street, Carlton
  Victoria 3053, Australia

Other Editorial Offices:
Arnette Blackwell SA
  1, rue de Lille, 75007 Paris
  France

Blackwell Wissenschafts-Verlag GmbH
  Kurfürstendamm 57
  10707 Berlin, Germany

  Feldgasse 13, A-1238 Wien
  Austria

First published 1989
Reprinted 1990 (twice), 1991
Second Edition 1995

Set in 11/13pt Times
by DP Photosetting, Aylesbury, Bucks
Printed and bound in Great Britain by
Hartnolls Ltd., Bodmin, Cornwall
Cover picture by Elizabeth Furth

DISTRIBUTORS

Marston Book Services Ltd
PO Box 87
Oxford OX2 0DT
(*Orders:* Tel: 01865 791155
       Fax: 01865 791927
       Telex: 837515)

USA
  Blackwell Science, Inc.
  238 Main Street
  Cambridge, MA 02142
  (*Orders:* Tel: 800 215-1000
         617 876-7000
         Fax: 617 492-5263)

Canada
  Oxford University Press
  70 Wynford Drive
  Don Mills
  Ontario M3C 1J9
  (*Orders:* Tel: 416 441-2941)

Australia
  Blackwell Science Pty Ltd
  54 University Street
  Carlton, Victoria 3053
  (*Orders:* Tel: 03 347-5552)

A catalogue record for this title
is available from the British Library

ISBN 0–632–03821–7

Library of Congress
Cataloging-in-Publication Data

Brown, Jeremy Houghton.
   Horse business management: managing a
successful yard/Jeremy Houghton Brown
and Vincent Powell-Smith. — 2nd ed.
     p. cm.
   Includes index.
   ISBN 0–632–03821–7
   1. Horse industry—Great Britain.
I. Powell-Smith, Vincent. II. Title.
HD9434.G72B76   1995
636.1'0068—dc20
                              95-5750
                              CIP

(M) 636.168 H.

Contents

Preface

This book is about good practice. To do things more efficiently and more effectively brings greater rewards; this is true both in running the horse business and in running the stable yard. Without losing traditional skills and standards, good management can bring greater success, however that is measured.

The horse industry now takes its rightful place alongside several others which are significant leaders in leisure and recreation. The government has a minister with special responsibility for our industry, and the European Union liaises over many matters. Tourists come from all over the world to enjoy this feature of Britain. In many rural areas it is a major employer and part of the fabric of our countryside.

Yet the horse industry is made up, for the most part, of small units: stable yards each with a few staff. Often there is a major personal commitment by the owner; the yard manager may also be working with a commitment which is rare in other industries. Staff and trainees alike show a zeal which stems from pride in their work and love for the horses in their care.

The aim of this book is to make every stable yard a more rewarding place and business – rewarding in terms of finance but also in terms of the pride engendered in all who work there. A prosperous and flourishing business is good news. A yard that is smart and happy is a joy to all who visit it or work in it.

The authors thank all who have advised on the contents of this book including Alastair Sutherland who has helped with the preparation of this second edition and particularly contributed to the section which deals with some management skills specified in National Vocational Qualifications.

The book unashamedly borrows much from other industries; it sets out ideas and methods that are well proven to bring good results.

Most yards practise excellent horse care. The aim of this book is to bring a parallel level of skill into the care of the business and all who work there.

1 Horses: a business and an industry

The horse industry and its organizations

'Horses' and 'industry' are not a contradiction in terms. An industry is a branch of commercial enterprise concerned with the output of a specified product or service. It is an organized economic activity, and in this sense the horse industry is a significant one in the UK. Because those who work with horses are not grouped into factories, found on industrial estates or located in the high street, it is easy to underestimate their number. The horse industry is fragmented but is a major employer of labour, though its identity and significance is often overlooked. This may be because of the small size and variety of the various individual units of which it is comprised.

Agriculture, in contrast, has long been accepted as a major industry. Successive governments have assigned ministers to watch over and help it, while the horse industry is left largely to fend for itself, despite the fact that, other than farming, it is the largest land-based industry; others are forestry, horticulture and fish-farming. However, the tide turned in 1987 when Mr Ted Smith, speaking for the government, said: 'There has been a change in policy; we now see a significant role for horses and intend to assist'. The following year the British Horse Society published a major report on the size of the British horse industry. It showed that there are:

- about half a million horses and ponies;
- three million regular riders;
- a total annual turnover of £760 million;
- £50 million exports;
- 800,000 hectares of land used for horses.

A survey conducted for *Horse and Hound* magazine in 1992 showed that 24 per cent of UK households claim some involvement with horses and 6 per cent of them claim to have a member of the household who rides. This survey estimated that the ancillary trades have a turnover of at least £350 million per annum. In 1994 the Royal Agricultural Society of England estimated that equine pursuits are growing at a rate of 4 per cent per annum.

It is possible to classify industries in many ways, ranging from numbers employed, capital employed, turnover, land use, foreign currency earnings to contribution in terms of pleasure or product. The horse industry scores highly under all these headings. Figures suggest that there are between 50,000 and 60,000 people working directly with horses as either employees or on a self-employed basis, but taking into account those indirectly involved – who range from farriers to bookmakers – this figure can be trebled. Indeed, in a House of Commons debate in 1984 it was stated that between 150,000 and 250,000 people were employed in the horse industry in its wider sense. Figure 1.1 is based on several sources

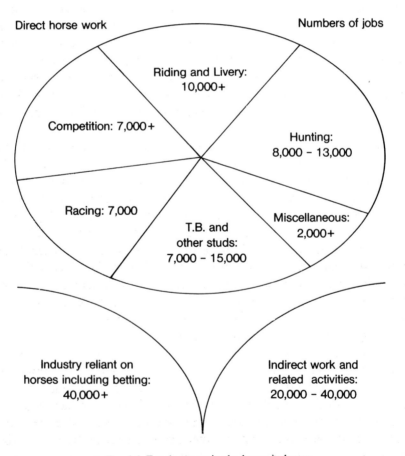

Fig. 1.1 Employment in the horse industry.

including the British Horse Society survey. Variations in the figures are due to seasonality, part-time workers and trainees.

The horse industry also has a diffuse image because it is divided into three parts:

- the racing industry;
- the non-thoroughbred industry;
- horse-associated activities.

The racing industry

The racing industry consists of breeding, rearing, buying and selling, and the training and racing of thoroughbred horses. It is sometimes called the thoroughbred industry and is divided into flat racing and National Hunt racing 'over the sticks'. It has a high profile and an enormous following. The horses are valuable and the prizes are large. The lucrative side of racing is flat racing, when young horses are trained to race as two- and three-year-olds. They may then be retired to stud, be culled or, more rarely, will stay in racing. There is a high wastage rate and of the mares going to a stallion, less than half will produce progeny that become race horses. The average two-year-old only races twice, and the average three-year-old only three times. It is a tough business and behind the glamour of the racecourse lie high risks.

National Hunt racing is divided into steeplechasing, hurdling and hunter chasing, of which steeplechasing and hurdling provide the majority of business for professional trainers. It is also a hard business, as it takes place through the autumn, winter and spring. Although the horses are tough and mature, they are subjected to the great stress of big jumps, high speeds, heavy weights and ground that may be deep or hard.

The British Horseracing Board is the governing body responsible for controlling flat racing and steeplechasing in Britain. The Jockey Club is the ruling body of the sport and has wide powers of discipline, including power to fine a trainer or jockey or to withdraw or suspend a licence to train or ride. The Jockey Club also lays down regulations for point-to-pointing, which is the amateur version of steeplechasing.

The breeding of racehorses is co-ordinated by the Thoroughbred Breeders Association, founded in 1917. Its objects are to encourage and ensure co-operative effort in all matters pertaining to the production and improvement of thoroughbred horses and the interests of their breeders.

Trainers come together under the National Trainers' Federation, which was formed to protect the interests of flat racing trainers. Stable lads (of both sexes) have a choice between the Stable Lads' Association or the Racing and Equestrian Section of the Agricultural and Allied Workers National Trade Group within the Transport and General Workers' Union.

Arab racing is another side of the racing industry. It is quite separate from flat and National Hunt racing, and is increasing in popularity. Harness racing is also distinct and is growing rapidly in popularity under the guidance of the British Harness Racing Club. In many parts of the world harness racing rivals gallop racing.

The non-thoroughbred industry

This is the largest section of the horse industry since it covers all others who have horses and ponies. It can be divided in various ways, such as breeders and users, but this is not really very helpful. The most logical method of classification is by organizations, because this is how the industry sees itself.

The largest and oldest part of this sector is hunting. The majority of packs of hounds hunt the fox (a few foxes are hunted on foot in mountain country). There are also harriers which hunt the hare (beagles also hunt hares but with both Hunt staff and followers on foot) and buck hounds and stag hounds hunt deer. Hunt followers subscribe to individual Hunts. The Masters of Foxhounds Association (MFHA), founded in 1881, stands in some respects in the same position to fox-hunting as the Jockey Club does to racing, but there is an important difference between the two organizations. The MFHA deals only with Masters of Foxhounds and committees of recognized Hunts; it has no control over individual fox-hunters. A recognized Hunt is one that has been officially accepted by the Committee of the MFHA and whose name is recorded on the official list of recognized Hunts.

Individual hunting folk belong to the British Field Sports Society, which is a strong and active body representative of all country sports and not merely of hunting.

Pleasure riders may well belong to a local Riding Club, which will probably be affiliated to the British Horse Society (BHS), which was founded in 1947 by the amalgamation of older organizations and which is now the authority and parent body of all horse and pony interests in Great Britain. Younger riders may well belong to their local branch of the Pony Club, which is also part of the BHS. Usually, each Pony Club is named after the local Hunt and has strong connections with it, but there is an increasing number of urban branches of the Pony Club where there is no Hunt.

Many people who ride each week do not have their own horse or pony and rely for their mounts on the local riding school. These establishments have to be licensed by the local authority, but may also be affiliated to the BHS and/or the Association of British Riding Schools (ABRS). Both of these organizations have a system of examinations for both pleasure and career riders. The National Pony Society (NPS), founded in 1893, also has an examination structure and offers training and qualifications in stud management. The NPS takes particular responsibility for Britain's native breeds. Show ponies, which are based on native breeds crossed with thoroughbred and Arab blood, are the concern of the British Show Pony Society. It is the controlling body for improving and regulating the showing of children's riding ponies. A third national pony society – the Ponies Association (UK) (formerly Ponies of Britain) – is particularly associated with showing. The British Horse Society also takes an interest in trekking, and there are other associations such as the Trekking and Riding Society of Scotland and the Scottish Trekking and Riding Association.

Another major group within the non-thoroughbred sector consists of competitive riders who are divided into various disciplines. In terms of both popularity and television coverage, show jumping is the most important competitive discipline. Clubs and riding schools organize jumping at local level, but the more serious contests are affiliated to the British Show Jumping Association (BSJA) which is the controlling body of show jumping in Great Britain. The BSJA is represented at international level by the British Equestrian Federation (BEF), which also represents the British Horse Society in international arrangements for dressage, horse trials, vaulting driving and long-distance riding. The BHS has separate groups for each of these sports. The British Driving Society is a specialist association for those interested in the driving of horses and ponies. There is also the Endurance Horse and Pony Society. The International Equestrian Federation (Fédération Equestre Internationale) governs the sport of riding on an international basis. It consists of representatives of the affiliated national bodies.

Polo stands alone as a sport, and is governed by the Hurlingham Polo Association which has jurisdiction over the game.

Competing includes showing, and every breed of horse has its own breed society. Various national bodies are concerned with breeds or types. These include the British Show Hack, Cob and Riding Horse Association, which was founded in 1938 to further the interests of owners and breeders of hacks and cobs; the National Light Horse Breeding Society (HIS), founded in 1885 to improve the type and promote the breeding of hunters and other riding horses; and the British Warm Blood Society founded in 1980. Many other societies exist to serve the needs of horse breeders. The British Horse Database, launched in 1993, exists to provide a comprehensive record of the parentage and progress of all horses and ponies in the UK; as with racing, this data is recorded by Wetherbys.

The thousands of horse and pony owners who merely ride for pleasure also form part of the non-thoroughbred sector. Many of them belong to the British Horse Society which tries to care for their interests. The final – and an important – group are disabled people who benefit in many ways from contact with horses. The Riding for the Disabled Association (RDA) was formed as a charity in 1969 to encourage riding for the physically and mentally disabled. Regional groups have been formed throughout the UK as well as in continental Europe.

The Equestrian Section of the Agricultural and Allied Workers Trade Group which is part of the Transport and General Workers' Union offers a trade union for all who work with horses. Its parent body offers a trade union for many who work in the horse-associated activities.

Horse-associated activities

The third sector of the horse industry consists of all those who rely partly or wholly on horses for a living. These associated activities include:

- veterinary surgeons;
- farriers and blacksmiths;
- auctioneers;
- knackers;
- saddlers and loriners;
- feed compounders and merchants;
- insurers and insurance agents;
- tack shops and horse clothiers;
- showground and racetrack staff;
- bookmakers and betting shops;
- horse society staff;
- sporting tailors and outfitters;
- bootmakers and hatters;
- journalists and publishers;
- cart and carriage makers;
- horsebox and trailer makers;
- stabling manufacturers and builders;

- hauliers and transporters;
- hunt staff;
- college staff;

and many others.

There are many specialist organizations representative of these various interests. These include, for example, the British Equine Veterinary Association, the Farriers Registration Council and the Society of Master Saddlers. There are related livery companies of the City of London such as the Worshipful Company of Loriners, the Worshipful Company of Saddlers and the Worshipful Company of Farriers.

An overall trade association is the British Equestrian Trade Association which holds trade fairs and publishes an excellent directory covering the whole of the horse industry and providing up-to-date names, addresses and telephone numbers, as well as an annual review of changes affecting the industry.

Because the horse industry is so diverse, ambitious school-leavers now can consider a broader list of possible horse careers than was formerly the case (Fig. 1.2).

- Manager, administrator, executive secretary
- Sales, marketing, technical and advisory officers
- Equestrian centre manager
- Stud manager, bloodstock agent
- Journalist, media work
- Public relations, communications
- Lecturer, instructor, coach
- Dealer, livery yard manager
- Stabling, transport, tack
- Health care, consultant
- Trainer, head girl, groom
- Rider, racing lad, driving

Fig. 1.2 Some jobs in the horse industry.

Training and education

In the early 1980s, the government appointed a committee under the chairmanship of Charles Ansell to investigate training and education leading to qualifications in the land-based industries. Its report (Report of the National Consultative Group for the Co-ordination of Validating Arrangements in Agriculture and Related Subjects) was published in 1985. The government initiative brought together the various horse associations concerned with training, and it was agreed to progress Ansell's recommendations before the publication of the final report. In 1983, a Working Group for Training and Education for work with horses was set up under the chairmanship of the late Dorian Williams. The Group set out to produce a ladder of skills for those seeking a career with horses, and published this as *Levels of Horse Care and Management*, Book 1 (1985) and Book 2 (1986). The principal authors were the late Pat Smallwood and Jeremy Houghton Brown; John Goldsmith of the BHS co-ordinated the work. Subsequently, the Group produced a *Directory of Career Training in the Horse Industry*. The Group's final task was to prepare the way for the Horse Council or the National Horse Education and Training Council (NHETC).

The NHETC was formed in 1987 to provide a forum for consultation between government, industry, education and training bodies on all aspects of education and training in the horse industry. Its logo is shown in Fig. 1.3. The NHETC was formed just at the right time because the government launched a programme of National Vocational Qualifications (NVQs) which required every industry to form its own 'lead body' and establish its own system of 'levels'. The horse industry was the only one in the country to have anticipated the need and to have already met both of these requirements.

The 'levels' are not examination syllabuses, but form a common standard available to all the examining bodies dealing with horses. To meet national requirements, the levels have to be expressed in a particular

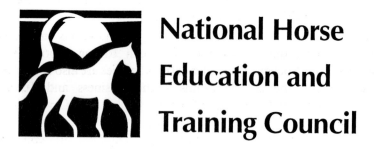

Fig. 1.3 The logo of the NHETC (from 1987 to 1995 it was called the Joint National Horse Education and Training Council (JNHETC)).

format which shows both the skills and the criteria for judging performance. In due course, all career qualifications awarded by all organizations will also be credited as NVQs. This should lead to:

'. . . development of a better trained, competent, qualified workforce; increased co-operation between employers, training organizations and awarding bodies; increased individual motivation and awareness of standards on the part of employees and easier identification and recruitment of competent staff'.

To meet NVQ requirements, examinations will be taken in units, bit by bit, and many will be tested at the workplace and not at an examination centre.

In Scotland there is a parallel system leading to Scottish Vocational Qualifications (SVQs).

The NHETC, then, is responsible for all aspects of training and education in the horse industry and for the maintenance of standards. It is recognized by the Training Commission as a 'non-statutory training organization' and 'industry-led body'. Much of its work has been in establishing levels for the National Council for Vocational Qualifications (NCVQ).

For use in schools and general technical colleges there is a system called General National Vocational Qualifications (GNVQs). These form alternatives to GCSEs and 'A' levels; they do not offer vocational competence.

For making comparison between different countries there is an International Group for Instructor Qualifications. They categorize these, and our BHSAI falls into their Level One, our BHSII into their Level Two and our BHSI into their Level Three.

The main horse organizations offering examinations are the British Horse Society, the Association of British Riding Schools and the National Pony Society. Two other national bodies are also concerned and these validate the college exams – the Business and Technology Education Council (BTEC) and City and Guilds. BTEC caters for those who are attending Agricultural or Technical Colleges for two or three years in order to gain a Diploma or Higher Diploma. Students working for City and Guilds examinations attend college for one year in order to gain a Certificate or Advanced Certificate. The professional horse management qualifications are shown in Fig. 1.4.

The one and two year 'Work Based Training' scheme, better known by its old title of 'Youth Training' (YT) scheme, is a recognized route of entry for a career in the horse industry. It is a scheme designed to prepare those

Levels		Societies				Examination bodies (college-based exams)	
Levels of horse care and management	NVQ Levels	British Horse Society Horsemastership	British Horse Society Teaching	Association of British Riding Schools	National Pony Society	City and Guilds	Business and Technology Education Council (BTEC)
1 Trainee	1	Horse Knowledge and Riding I	—	Preliminary Horse Care and Riding I	Stud Trainee Certificate Part I	—	—
2 Competent worker (needs supervision)	2	Horse Knowledge and Riding II	—	Preliminary Horse Care and Riding II	Stud Trainee Certificate Part II	—	—
3 Competent (can use initiative and can supervise)	3	Horse Knowledge and Riding III / ASSISTANT INSTRUCTOR	Preliminary Teaching Certificate	Assistant Groom Certificate	Stud Assistant Certificate	National Certificate in the Management of Horses	BTEC General and Business Studies (Horse) Diploma
4 Manager	4	Horse Knowledge and Riding IV / INTERMEDIATE INSTRUCTOR / Stable Management Certificate Equitation + Teaching / INSTRUCTOR	Intermediate Teaching Certificate	Groom's Diploma / Riding School Principal's Diploma	Stud Diploma / Stud Manager's Diploma	Advanced National Certificate in Equine Business Management / —	BTEC Horse Studies and Management Diploma / BTEC Higher National Diploma in Horse Studies (Management and Technology)

Fig. 1.4 Professional horse management qualifications.

Notes:
(1) It may be appropriate to take more than one qualification at any level.
(2) The college-based exams at any level tend to include in the course of study considerable preparation for the next level up.

leaving school for the world of work and is available to those aged 16 and older. It combines working in a yard for a 'work experience provider' (WEP), with attendance at a college or training centre on a day release or block release basis. Trainees are encouraged to take examinations which lead to recognized qualifications. The scheme is organized and co-ordinated by local Training and Enterprise Councils (TECs) acting through agent organizations.

An advantage of YT as a system of formal training is that it is monitored by all sides of industry to ensure that employers (as work experience providers) adhere to the conditions of the scheme. It is not intended to be a form of cheap labour. YT is government-sponsored. The trainee receives a weekly allowance and this is payable even when the trainee is on holiday. The WEP is expected to make a financial contribution. The trainee works a 40 hour week. Overtime is not compulsory, but if performed by the trainee must be paid for at a realistic rate. The trainee is entitled to 26 days' holiday each year. These conditions came as something of a shock to many people engaged in the horse industry where, on the thoroughbred side, the working week is about 40 to 46 hours, and on the non-thoroughbred side is typically between 50 and 60 hours.

Initial training and education is the right way to start a career and leads to jobs and ongoing education and training. The horse industry has yet to achieve a clear career structure with good opportunities for the most able. To some extent, this exists in the thoroughbred sector, but the lack of such a structure on the non-thoroughbred side leads to an enormous wastage of young people leaving the industry and to a shortage of well-qualified and experienced staff. The developments now taking place at national level should do much to combat this.

Choice of enterprise and management style

There are many types of business within the horse industry, and within each business there may be several different enterprises. An enterprise in this sense is a unit within the business as a whole – a riding school may offer livery as well as buying and selling horses and ponies. The difficulty lies not so much in the choice of enterprise, but in deciding why that enterprise is a sensible venture. Many horse businesses continue for years without any reappraisal of the situation, and many people start a horse business without reviewing all the possibilities.

Selecting the right enterprise calls for self-examination about one's motives and ambitions. 'What am I seeking to achieve in my life?' is the sort of question to be asked. An honest answer would in general be a mixture of 'Take pride in all I do', 'Achieve something worthwhile' and 'Follow my star'!

A love of animals may give one the ambition to become a veterinary surgeon, but despite hard work and good motivation, the necessary exceptional 'A' level grades may not be achieved. Such a person might find a closely-related career with animals satisfying and rewarding, perhaps in the horse industry. Another person who was attracted to horses may have spent most of their spare time riding, caring for horses or perhaps even just thinking about them, but performed badly in school examinations, left as soon as possible, and then embarked on a career with horses. Thus people come into the industry by different routes, and in due course come to the point of deciding what enterprise they wish to manage or business they wish to create. The basic criteria are straightforward. One should concentrate on what one does best. The criterion of

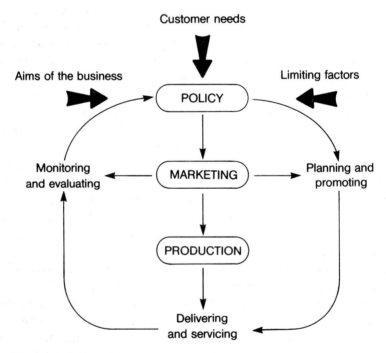

Of the three main management responsibilities, Policy, Marketing and Production, many horse businesses concentrate on the third almost to the exclusion of the other two and greatly to the detriment of the business

Fig. 1.5 The management of a business.

pride is more demanding; it may seek profit for a desired lifestyle; it may seek success in competition or through reputation. Satisfying it will require that the chosen business is well-run and is profitable.

To achieve these objectives requires an amalgam of wise decisions: good location, suitable aims and good management.

There are many styles of management, and these are best considered separately. The management of a business is shown in Fig. 1.5.

Management by objectives

In a large company, the board of directors usually establishes a long-term plan and short-term objectives, and the company's performance is monitored. Where there has been under-performance, the underlying reasons will be analysed and the plan reviewed. If good performance is achieved, the success is analysed and new targets are set. Long-term objectives will change in the light of the political and financial climates, the activities of competitors, and technological and other changes.

A sales company, for example, will have a national sales target, which will be divided into regional figures which regional sales managers are realistically expected to achieve. The regions will be divided into areas with each area manager having a target, and in turn the individual salesmen's targets will be set. The company's overall objective is thus divided and each individual is under pressure to help to achieve it. Bonuses may be offered to individuals and all those involved have a corporate desire to achieve their individual targets.

Few businesses in the horse industry set such specific targets; pipe-dreams seem to be more the order of the day. But successful businesses do set objectives. A riding school might set the target of achieving a 20 per cent increase in the number of lessons given by a stated date. A stud could plan to achieve a 15 per cent higher price for its yearlings than was the case the previous year.

Targets can be published and discussed, but they must be realistically achievable and the management must be able to show the staff that this is the case. A riding school teacher might, for example, say that he/she could attract more clients if only the school was not so dusty, the noise of passing traffic did not drown his/her instruction or if parents did not get so cold while waiting. These are long-standing and well-known problems at the school, but with a set target and staff involvement, the teacher's problems are clearly identified as the stumbling blocks to the achievement of the objective. In this light, possible solutions can be costed and the costs compared against the likely or possible increase in business.

If a manager is to achieve the owner's objectives, these must be spelt out and given a time-scale. A manager's hardest task is often to find out exactly what the owner wants from the business. The honest answer may be that the owner wants to give the business to a daughter five years hence as a thriving concern. At first sight, such an answer might be thought to demotivate the manager, but in fact the manager should be delighted to face such a clear-cut challenge to his/her ability. In five years time, the business should be so buoyant and have such high standards and well-trained staff that its new owner can take over. The business would maintain the manager's style and the staff would have the continuing pleasure of working in a happy and prosperous environment. With such success behind the manager, he/she would find other establishments clamouring for his/her services if the new owner wished to manage the concern herself and had the ability to do so.

If the owner or manager is to keep the policy for the business up-to-date the following options must be considered:

(a) What future changes may occur to the situation?
    What are the probabilities of these changes happening?
    What would be the consequences of these changes?

(b) What are the business's strengths?
    What are its weaknesses?
    What savings could be made?
    What new projects or enterprises could be created?
    What threats does the future hold?

Management for quality

It is not easy to make a profit from running a horse business. Many horse businesses are family concerns which utilize the home and the time of all the family to achieve pleasure but not much profit. Others start out in high hopes and with a heavy mortgage, but the competition is too stiff and the owners quit the struggle. But in every area of the country there tends to be a horse business – stud, livery yard or riding school – which becomes *the* place to go to from the clients' point of view. Usually, the common factor is *quality*. Achieving it is not simply a matter of decision by the owners. Quality is only achieved by getting commitment from staff and this means offering them responsibility. Overall commitment to quality and the achievement of set objectives is clearly demonstrated by Japanese industrial companies which adopt a 'total team' approach to success, and the same principles can be applied to any business.

Staff and clients alike enjoy associating with a business which has a reputation for quality. Pride and morale rise. People like to do things well. Quality involves a commitment to the clients and the more a business commits itself to clients, the more they will commit themselves to the business. As one successful event rider said: 'When I need a new young horse I always go back to the same dealer. Although I have to pay a little more for the horse, over the years I have always found it good value'.

Management by organization

Any business, however small, must be organized yet some businesses appear to be organized chaos. At one riding school, for example, when sufficient clients have arrived at the yard, they go with their instructor to catch their horses. Lessons are held in open fields amongst grazing horses. The horses are turned loose afterwards, the clients pay the instructor in cash, which the instructor places in an urn in the hall of the owner's house. The local farmer delivering hay is paid from the same urn.

Generally a horse business will have a clear chain of command but if they are only commands dissatisfaction will ensue. The better character-istics to look for are specialization in particular jobs which are ongoing posts in that business so suitably qualified individuals can be recruited; thus the business has or trains up the best people for the jobs. Secondly the hierarchy of authority is clear and includes responsibility at every level. Dissatisfaction is inevitable if the head lad gives an order and two minutes later the trainer arrives in the yard and countermands that order. Such problems are particularly prevalent when there is an owning family and a manager: the poor manager finds his staff receiving conflicting instructions from different members of the family.

It follows that the organization must have rules; rules for safety are obvious, though sometimes overlooked. Rules about agreed procedures are essential. Some procedures may be complex, e.g. those in case of fire, while others are simple routines such as how a stranger is to be greeted if found in the yard, or how telephone enquiries should be dealt with. Some rules must be worked out carefully; for example, agreement with the vet and the stud groom as to the procedure for the person sitting up when a mare goes into labour.

Another characteristic of a successful organization is that the format is not built around individual personality and preference but around achieving the agreed set objectives. Individual personalities can be a wonderful asset and it would be foolish to ignore special skills, but a successful business does not redirect its activities to fall in with the wishes of its staff.

The formal organization of a business is not bureaucratic and impersonal. A carefully-defined and orderly organization allows for equality of treatment because it is rational. The problem is one of balance. The organization should not be inflexible, neither should it be so formal that loyalty is lost.

In larger companies lines of responsibility are often based on what is called 'the rule of five'. This states that no person should be responsible for or supervise any more than five direct subordinates. Thus, the owner of a riding school may have up to five key people each charged with responsibility for an area: the yard manager, the chief instructor, the secretary and the estate man, for example. Under some of these there may be a team of up to five assistants. The important point is that each individual must know to whom they are responsible and whom they should approach in case of doubt or difficulty. The key concept is a team which understands and cares for the job and whose members care for each other.

The manager receives the highest remuneration because his/her decisions are crucial to the success or failure of the operation. When reaching a decision, good managers sound out the team and explain the position. Staff in general appreciate a manager's right to manage, but they also appreciate being kept in the picture. Good communications are a priority and must be built into the work routine and become a second habit. There must always be a time and place when staff can find out what is going on.

Managers have key responsibilities in the areas of administration, production and marketing. The last named is the area most commonly neglected in the horse world.

Management for profit

Profit is one of the most obvious but elusive indicators of success in managing a horse business. Professionals who are concerned with this aspect of the business include the bank manager and accountant whose livelihoods are largely provided by successful businesses.

The first essential is to know how the business is doing financially at present so that the true financial picture can be assessed. It is also useful to compare the position with that of other businesses of similar scope and size. Those who invest in a business – its owners and possibly their relatives as well as the bank – wish to know the return on their investment. A financial health-check of this kind shows up any areas of weakness.

If changes are planned, they must be budgeted for. Good records are essential, and the importance of proper financial management cannot be overstressed. Finance and profit are discussed in Chapter 6.

Marketing

Market-orientated management is probably the unrecognized philosophy behind many successful horse businesses. Marketing has been defined as 'producing a product that does not come back for customers who do' and is as much applicable to horse businesses as to any other.
    Marketing activities include:

- identifying the customer's requirement;
- gearing the business to satisfy the requirement and making a profit;
- reacting to change in customers' needs so that the business continues to be profitable;
- advertising and selling.

The product may be a horse, a breeding policy, a stallion at stud, a clipping service, a livery business – in fact, anything relating to horses.

A marketing campaign

Successful marketing requires a campaign. The elements of a campaign are easy to identify:

(1) *Find the idea.* This entails research by reading about new developments, attending conferences and visiting leading establishments. In this way one finds the market opportunity.
(2) *Consider the market.* Analyse the market and potential competition as well as the cost factors.
(3) *Prepare a plan.* In some cases it may be possible to run a pilot scheme or a test marketing exercise. Many possibilities are rejected at this stage.
(4) *Prepare for implementation.* An advertising and public relations campaign may be initiated and the media involved.
(5) *Launch the product.* Selling is an essential part of any business, but the entrepreneur must ensure that the necessary back-up can be provided. There is nothing to be gained and a great deal to be lost by advertising a service that cannot be provided. Customers simply go to someone who comes up with the goods. This amounts to advertising for a competitor.

(6) *Monitor on-going performance*, including quality control. Performance monitoring extends to advertising as well. It is an excellent
idea to ask every client how they first heard of the business. If nobody
mentions a particular publication it is probably not worth advertising
in it again. Examples of this can be seen in the trade press; clients are
asked to reply to Department XY. It is likely that XY is specific to
advertisements in one publication.

Experience is a learning process and may mean changes in plans. There
must be an awareness of changing market needs and a willingness to
adapt.

Other considerations include the owner's ambitions, staff competence,
training and needs, as well as the activities of competitors. There may be
various limiting factors too, such as locality or space.

Advertising

Advertising requires a systematic approach. In order to provide value for
money it must be based on research so that it is properly aimed and takes
any competition into account. The benefits of the product must be listed
and placed in order of importance so that the 'advertising message' is
clear. A campaign is then prepared to a budget and the advertisements are
drafted. A good advertisement meets four criteria of the acronym AIDA:

- Attracts attention.
- Interest is aroused.
- Desire is created.
- Action is stimulated.

A good advertisement thus catches the reader's eye and is immediately
interesting. The message stimulates a desire for the product. A good
advertisement should also stimulate immediate action, which accounts
for some of the success of mail-order selling.

Promotions

Public relations is an important aspect of any business (Fig. 1.6). It starts
with first impressions when a telephone enquiry is made. The first
impression is based on the way in which the telephone is answered and the
call is dealt with. Similarly, a prompt response to a letter and good
notepaper suggest quality, style and efficiency. Every business should
develop a 'house style' covering every detail: the notice boards, the colour

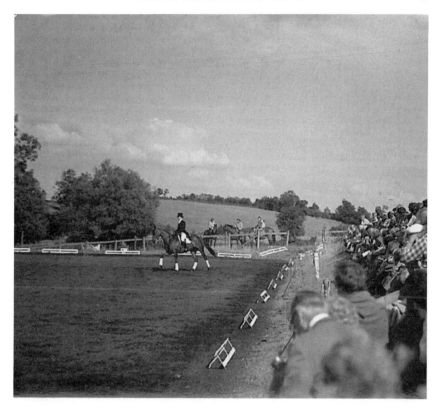

Fig. 1.6 An open day at a training centre is good for local public relations and also good publicity.

of the stable doors, notepaper, advertisements and press releases. This may extend to clothing for staff and horses or to the colour of horsebox or trailer. Having established a 'brand image' it is important to protect it. The lorry should be clean and the staff polite and efficient.

A new product may call for a launch combining several methods of promotion. A typical launch will have a guest speaker or celebrity to open the new building, welcome the new stallion or whatever. Media representatives and other guests will be invited and the budget must include refreshments. A press release should be prepared and distributed to the equestrian and local press and to local radio and television. The publicity obtained in this way can be far more effective than paid advertisements, but normally a campaign will combine both methods.

There are also opportunities for direct mail. Local equestrian organizations may be prepared to include a leaflet in their mailing to members in return for a contribution towards postage. Relevant directories and trade

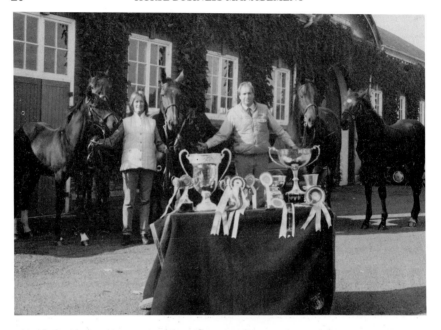

Fig. 1.7 Success in the show ring can increase the value of young stock sold from the stud; also it publicizes and increases the value of the stallions.

lists (as well as the Yellow Pages of the Telephone Directory) can form the basis of lists for direct mail. With new products aimed nationally, specialist promotion companies can be used, though their charges tend to be expensive.

A trade stand at a local show can pay dividends and attract new customers The exact nature and extent of the promotion will depend on the type of enterprise.

Care with the entry in the Telephone Directory, the Yellow Pages and Thompsons Directory is important. For riding schools and trekking centres a brochure or card can be placed in local leisure centres, inns, restaurants, libraries, hotels, guest houses and so on; also tourist information publications offer good possibilities. Showing is an important way of promoting a stud (Fig. 1.7). Stallions can be paraded at local shows and point-to-points. Competing, providing it is successful, is also useful and the horsebox acts as a publicity medium. Going hunting is an important means of making contacts in any area.

In summary, successful management requires clear objectives, quality, efficient organization, proper financial control and good marketing. The entrepreneur should check the business regularly against these criteria.

2 Premises

The site

The right location is important for any business and many factors must be taken into account when choosing a site. In many cases, there is no option of choice, since the site is already an established one. However, the considerations guiding someone who has the choice of location for a new horse enterprise are just as useful to those with an established business or for whom the location is already fixed.

Local topography is important – accessibility, centres of population, available resources and possible future developments are all factors which should be taken into account. For example, if the business is to be based on the giving of hourly riding lessons, by allowing for the quality of the lessons and the riders' level of expertise, the number of potential clients can be predicted. Beginners and those being instructed on a weekly basis will not wish to travel too far. In all probability, they will not drive past another riding school offering a similar service unless there is a strong incentive to do so.

Thus, when considering the suitability of premises for such a business, important questions are: 'Where are the clients?', 'How easy is it for them to get to lessons?' and 'Where is the competition?' Most riding schools need a nearby town in order to be successful. A business based on day-treks throughout the year will, in contrast, need three urban centres within an hour's drive.

As the product on offer becomes more specialized, people will travel further; a top-class dressage trainer may attract customers willing to travel several hours for a single lesson. If the enterprise is a stud standing several stallions, the questions must be 'Where are the mare owners?' and 'What other stallions are at stud in the district?' Owners will bring a mare a long way to the right stallion, but they appreciate a location convenient to the motorway network for fast and easy travel. A racehorse trainer must look to where potential patrons live; ideally, this should not be too

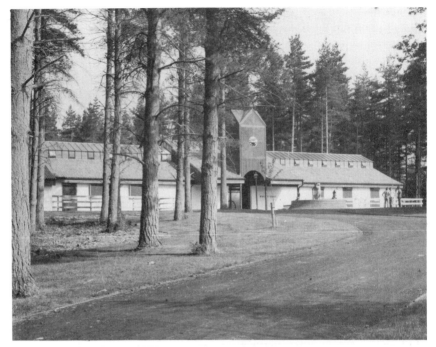

Fig. 2.1 A modern complex in southern England built for a royal Arab owner.

close but should be within range of visiting the stables. Racing stables need to be convenient to several racecourses and must be well served by major roads if the horses are to race further afield regularly.

After access, competition and customers, it is important to investigate the facilities available in the area. A trekking business needs bridleways that link up to create a variety of day-treks. A racing trainer will need gallops. Most horse activities benefit from quiet country lanes with wide grass verges. People getting horses fit, whether for hunting or competition, will need a few hills. Show jumpers should study the locations of the bigger indoor schools which are part of the winter show-jumping circuit.

However, it is important to look to the future. A proposed motorway coming close by will push up the value of a property dramatically, but one coming too close will depress its value and possibly cause cessation of business. Purchasing a property convenient to a famous dressage trainer is splendid for the dressage rider until the trainer moves away and the property is bought by a show jumping trainer! An area that seems to be crying out for a good riding school may seem an excellent place to buy a smallholding suitable for conversion – until one discovers, after buying the property, that a nearby farmer has obtained planning permission to convert his beef-fattening complex into a riding school. He has not only land and buildings which are easily convertible to stables and an indoor school, but may possibly have grant aid to establish his new business. Some of these problems are imponderable; others can be avoided by making local enquiries before agreeing to buy.

Soil type is also important for equine businesses. Ideally, the soil should be free-draining so as to allow some horses to be wintered out with consequent savings in labour and bedding. The free draining soils are generally those with a higher percentage of sand when compared with clay. They are generally called light soils or light land, not because of their weight but because they could be worked with a lighter team of horses. Loam – a mixture of sand, silt and clay – is what to look for. Heavier land, which is mostly clay, drains less well and so tends to get poached in winter and thus will not take horses from Christmas until it dries out in late spring. Heavy clay soils – even with drains – get deep and muddy in winter. Even in summer, heavier land can be difficult as, during a dry spell, it sets rock-hard and cracks. Farmers like heavier soils because they are more fertile and grow better crops, whereas light land is not only less productive but also feels the effects of drought more quickly and so may run short of grass in midsummer.

Land prices are another factor to be considered when selecting an area. In areas of high employment and prosperity, land tends to be more expensive than in less affluent areas. Hill land is cheaper than prime arable or pasture land. Milk and corn are the two main profit sources for most British farms and so land which is suitable only for beef and sheep will cost less. However, the initial price is only part of the picture. In many cases it will be more prudent to take a bigger mortgage on a more expensive property than to buy a cheap property with a low earning potential. Land prices rose rapidly for a decade, peaking in 1984, and then, due to decreasing farm profitability, steadied on a plateau before falling in the general recession. By 1994 they were climbing back towards the plateau, but may take some years to do so. Rents have followed a similar pattern. Term dates for tenancies vary with area and type of farming; common dates are Candlemas (2 February), Lady Day (25 March) and Michaelmas (29 September).

Planning and building regulations permission

Where there is already an established commercial horse business on a property, planning permission is probably unnecessary. However, this is one of the things that a solicitor should check when acting for a purchaser. Planning permission is needed for any 'development' and this includes what the planners call 'a material change of use', even if no building work is needed to carry out the change of use. Thus, planning permission will be required if private stabling is to be turned into a riding school or other commercial enterprise. Similarly, under the present law, if the established use is farming, planning permission will be needed if the use is to be changed to that of a horse business. Forms can be obtained from the local district council. If planning permission is refused at local level, the planning authority should tell you why and you may discuss the reasons with them and find out if their objections can be overcome. There is a right to appeal to the Secretary of State for the Environment, which may involve a public inquiry. If planning permission is required, it is sensible to engage the services of a local architect or chartered surveyor.

The planning authority's concerns are as follows:

- the provision of development plans for their area;
- the suitability of the site (and whether an alternative site may be available);
- the impact on the character or amenity value of the area;
- any employment considerations (show these as benefits);
- implications for volume and type of traffic, access and road safety;
- drainage and the burden on mains water and sewerage;
- appearance and materials used;
- effects on wildlife and landscape;
- noise, pollution and other nuisance.

Merely using land for grazing horses is regarded as an agricultural use and so planning permission is unnecessary. Individual private householders are also able to carry out certain 'permitted developments' without making an application for planning permission: erecting a stable or loose box is permitted and is regarded as the enlargement of the house itself. However, neither of these concessions is of much assistance to someone wishing to operate a horse business, and the question of planning permission (or lack of it) is an important factor when making a decision whether or not to acquire a property. An existing planning permission may lay down special conditions, and in National Parks, Areas of Outstanding Natural Beauty and conservation areas, there may be special restrictions.

Even if planning permission exists or is granted, building regulations approval must be sought if any structural work or work involving a change in the use of the premises is to be undertaken subject to minor

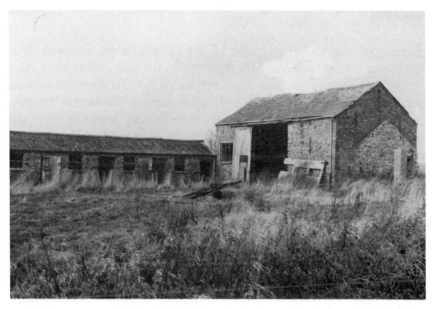

Fig. 2.2 Old premises suitable for conversion to private houses with stables now fetch high prices in many areas.

exceptions, e.g. approval is not needed to erect a small detached building of less than 30 square metres floor area, with no sleeping accommodation, such as a garden shed. The building regulations are administered by the building control officers of the district councils, from whom the appropriate forms are obtained. If unauthorized work is carried out, the district council can require its removal or alteration, but in practice if more than a year has elapsed since the work was completed, there is little they can do. Obtaining approval under the building regulations is not as difficult as obtaining planning permission, and local building control officers are generally most helpful.

Anyone intending to carry on the business of keeping horses either for the purpose of letting them out on hire and/or giving riding instruction for payment will require a Riding Establishment Licence from the district council. The present position in England, Wales and Scotland is governed by the Riding Establishments Acts 1964 and 1970, and is explained in Chapter 5. The law is under review and there is a lobby seeking to introduce changes such as raising the minimum age of those left in charge of the establishment and possibly of extending the legislation to include livery stables.

Suitability

When considering the purchase of an existing horse business, it is important to find out why the business is for sale. There may be a straightforward reason such as retirement or moving from the area or purchasing another enterprise. On the other hand, it may be that the seller has failed to make a profit. If this is so, there are two problems. First, the business may not be viable – at least in its present form. Second, the establishment may have earned itself a poor reputation. That may be more of a hindrance than having no reputation at all.

Working out whether premises are suitable is not an easy task. It requires a great deal of hard work in terms of planning, budgeting and costing. Even if the business can be established within one's available and procurable finances, there are still risks because the number of clients and the profitability of the business are largely conjectural in the case of a new business. Indeed, even when purchasing an established business with existing clients as a 'going concern' the same problem must be faced.

In some cases, one already has suitable premises to hand. The question then is 'Should we operate a horse business here and, if so, what sort of horse business should it be?' This question is not easy to answer, but experienced advice is available from various bodies. The government offers help through ADAS (Woodthorne, Wergs Road, Wolverhampton, West Midlands WV6 8TQ). The advice is not free, but the ADAS service offers good value for money, especially about problems which are similar to those in agriculture such as buildings, finance and land management.

The British Horse Society is a source of advice for its members. It publishes many specialist leaflets on common problems and offers good local contact and hence local specialist knowledge. Similarly, the Association of British Riding Schools offers help to those going into that area. The National Pony Society, the National Light Horse Breeding Society (HIS) and the Thoroughbred Breeders' Association are all able to assist those contemplating setting up stud farms. Horses are now within the scope of the Rural Development Agency. This body is an excellent source of advice and guidance on financial matters, grants available, training possibilities and marketing.

Finally, when considering suitability, the checklist should include:

- pleasing locality;
- access to main services;
- free-draining land;
- a southerly aspect;

- good safe hacking;
- tolerant neighbours.

Layout and principles

To some extent existing buildings dictate the overall layout, but they do not necessarily control it. The need may be for good lateral thinking. An existing building which at first sight appears crucial to the layout of the new buildings may in fact be better off demolished! The gap so created opens up a range of possibilities. When designing the layout is the time to be brave and resolute and look to the future. Those working in the yard later may condemn the lack of vision or the expediency which resulted in a poorly sited tack room. Good layout is a good investment in equine, human and financial terms.

There are no tested standard plans as there are in some areas of agriculture such as the layout of milking parlours and of yards leading to the cow cubicles and silage area. There are five criteria to bear in mind:

- Is it right for the horses?
- Is it right for those who work there?

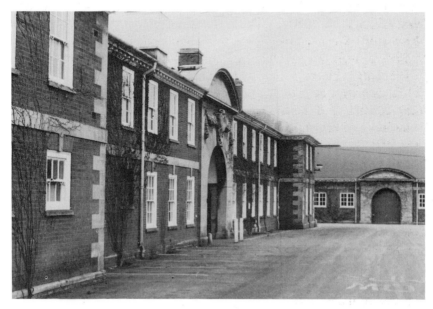

Fig. 2.3 Stabling, indoor school and accommodation built early this century to a standard which would now be prohibitively expensive.

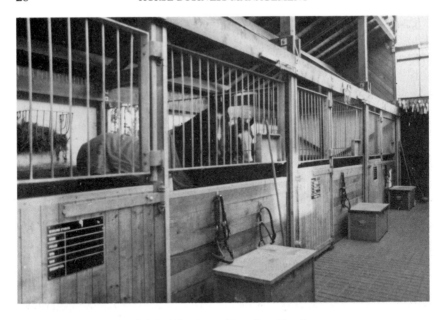

Fig. 2.4 Stabling in an 'American Barn' system.

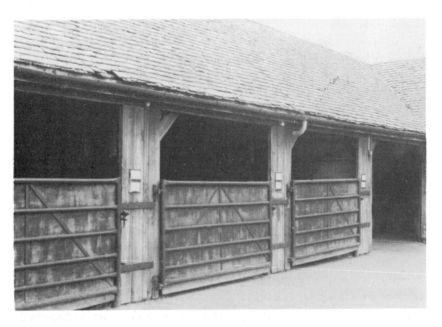

Fig. 2.5 Old cart sheds simply converted to make excellent stables.

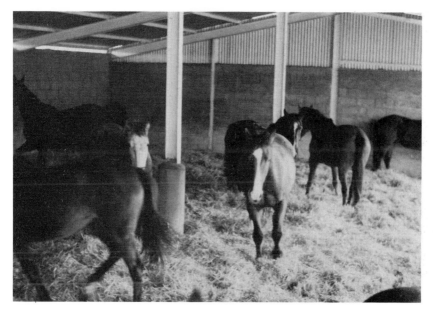

Fig. 2.6 Young horses winter well in barns.

- Is it right for clients?
- Is it aesthetically pleasing?
- Is it safe?

In balancing these criteria, the horses must come first. The range of possibilities is greater than at first appears. The housing for horses round the world shows a wide variation within the good results group. It is erroneous to attribute a human outlook to animals and hence it is a mistake to say 'Well, how would you like to live in a ...?'

Horses have a different attitude to their environment from that of human beings. They need plenty of fresh air and that is certainly missing from many stables. Bad stables have low roofs, no high outlet for stale air, poor air circulation and in some cases they even lack an inlet for fresh air. Horses need personal space in which to live without threat from a neighbour. This does not mean that stalls are necessarily bad, but it does mean that loose boxes with feed mangers facing each other through bars are.

Horses also need a regular and peaceful environment free from tension. This may be found in an old stone-built yard with doves, but it may equally be provided in a modern yard with pop music! Peace is disturbed by grooms who are tense or cross, irregular routines, sudden noises and events which are out of the ordinary. It is also disturbed by visitors who want to stroke the horses. Horses also need comfortable bedding, adequate food and water and regular exercise. This last feature is of particular importance in overall design which may include horse walkers, treadmills, maneges, indoor schools and exercise yards. All these things take up large areas of space and are thus key features in designing the layout.

Consideration for the people who will work in the yard and care for the horses is also essential when planning the layout. 'Work study' is the examination of ways of finding the best and most efficient method of doing a job, especially in terms of time and effort. In our context, it is especially concerned with the route taken during the daily routines – morning and evening stables, tacking up and other regular tasks. Good layout can shorten the route and thus save time, effort and expense. Sometimes putting in a door or relocating the muck heap can make a great deal of difference to the daily life of a groom. Good design reduces drudgery and increases effectiveness.

Major decisions about the style of housing should be strongly influenced by considerations of the employee, so they should be consulted. One of the main reasons for stabling horses in barns is that it is quicker and easier for the grooms as well as being tidier than a row of loose boxes. The same argument applies to the use of stalls. Mares in stalls provide the speediest way of mucking out a large number of horses. A good drain will already have coped with the urine, the faeces are conveniently placed to load into the barrow and the bedding stays dry and needs little attention. Geldings are less helpful; they wet their bedding.

All stabling should look good and be appropriate to its function and to the site. Architects are often criticized for creating new designs which look out of place against existing buildings. In some cases, the criticism is well-founded; in others, the real criticism was that the offence was caused by the new building being 'different', and in retrospect has in fact blended in quite well. Colours, shapes, texture of materials, the outline from different viewpoints and first impressions are all important considerations. In many cases, the additional cost may prevent one from using the more expensive materials; the good use of colour and careful landscaping can make cheaper materials quite as acceptable.

Moving earth to make banks can provide screens against prying eyes, wind and sound. Planned planting of trees, shrubs and creepers at the building stage can rapidly make a great improvement to the visual appearance of the premises. In the same way, good use of colour and choice of materials can vastly improve the interior of a building without any great increase in the overall cost. Design is the function of architects whose education prepares them to assist clients at all stages of the design and construction process, but the architect's client must provide adequate information on the site, project and budget, and fully understand and approve the architect's proposals at each stage. The client must be able to brief the architect adequately if the architect is to perform his/her professional functions properly. Both employees and clients will appreciate a stable block built with thought for its layout and aesthetic appearance.

Safety is the fourth criterion in layout. It is a major factor because of one's legal and moral responsibilities towards employees and members of the public. Safety is very important in riding schools or any other premises to which the public has access. In a riding school, for example, the design should provide for visitors to go directly to a reception or waiting area, thus avoiding the risk of their poking around the yard, upsetting the horses and causing an accident. In a stud, the layout will concentrate on the stallions which tend to be more peaceful if mares are not led past their boxes. Someone could be grooming a stallion when an in-season mare is led past and both groom and the mare's handler would then be put at risk. Good design takes such things into account. Figure 2.7

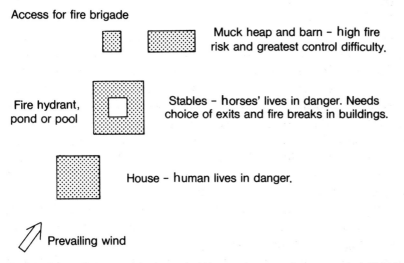

Design to cope with fire

Access for fire brigade

Muck heap and barn – high fire risk and greatest control difficulty.

Fire hydrant, pond or pool

Stables – horses' lives in danger. Needs choice of exits and fire breaks in buildings.

House – human lives in danger.

Prevailing wind

Fig. 2.7 Areas of greatest risk: downwind. Areas of greatest danger: upwind. This design also keeps the 'dust' from the barns away from the stables, thus aiding horse health.

shows how a fire travelling with the prevailing wind moves away from the area of greatest danger and is an example of good design. Some horses are very protective of their feed to an extent which makes them difficult at feed time, especially if they have not been taught good stable manners. Feed mangers in the far corner of stables are not only a waste of time; they also can create tension between horse and groom, and where there is tension there is danger. Mangers filled from outside are both quicker and safer.

Small, placid ponies do well in covered straw yards. Bigger horses and cobs prosper in stalls, but need daily exercise. Horses that have a stand-in day (when they are not exercised) as part of the weekly routine need to be in loose boxes. (Stand-in days only benefit employees; horses do better without them.) Thoroughbred mares have been wintered successfully in stalls when exercised daily on a horse-walker. Tense and highly-strung horses do better in loose boxes, which can be in barns or set around a yard. The cost difference between loose boxes and stalls is less than the range of prices within each system – quality buildings are always expensive.

The many items to include in a complete stable yard are shown in Table 2.1.

Table 2.1 Requirements of a stable yard.

(1) Loose boxes	(17) Locker and changing room
(2) Stalls	(possibly with shower)
(3) Stock yards	(18) Staff lounge
(4) Feed room	(19) Store – for paint, lawnmower,
(5) Hay store	etc.
(6) Straw or bedding store	(20) Garages and parking areas for
(7) Bulk or back-up feed store	horsebox, tractor, staff, visitors
(8) Wash area: buckets, rugs, etc.	(21) Wheelbarrow park
(9) Wash area: horses	(22) Fire and security control
(10) Drying room	points
(11) Dirty tack cleaning area	(23) Clock
(12) Clean tack store	(24) Isolation box
(13) Utility box (clipping, heat	(25) Specialist stud units, e.g. stallion
lamp)	quarters, foaling unit, covering
(14) Manure bunker	and teasing yard
(15) Office	(26) Forge
(16) Lavatory	(27) Mounting block

Detail design

The guiding principles of detail design are that the end result should be safe, functional and labour-saving. For example, a manger which can be filled from outside the loose box is a simple essential if employees are to be well-paid and cost-effective; this can be achieved with a manger on a tilt, swivel or hinge system or with a trap door above it of sufficient size to allow for the feed bucket. Similarly, the hay rack should be filled from outside; this not only saves time but, because the rack is filled from the side and not the top, also allows for the rack to be lower in the stable and to be fitted with a mesh lid to prevent the horse lifting the hay out of the top. The lower fitting is better for the horse because it is less likely to get a grass seed in its eye; it is also better for the person whose job it is to fill the hay racks.

Automatic drinkers are another time-saving essential. Such devices have an unjustifiably bad reputation but most problems can be solved by installing them correctly. The supply tank should be fitted in the roof so that the system is gravity-fed rather than fed direct from the mains. The supply line should be fitted with a tap to each drinker, thus enabling ease of adjustment and maintenance. A drain cock must be fitted at the lowest point so that during very cold weather the system can be drained off each evening to avoid overnight freezing. There must also be a well-insulated tap for use during very cold periods. This water tap is best sited in the feed room, preferably over a big Belfast-style sink set near to the floor. The sink unit serves for washing buckets in an ordinary routine. Each stable needs a tie ring near the hay rack and another well away from it. Each tie ring should be fitted with a loop of parcel string or strong garter elastic (*not* plastic bale twine) so as to provide a weakest link to break if there is a fracas, so avoiding a broken head collar or the tie ring being pulled from the wall. When training horses to be tied up, a long line running through a strong ring or around a post or tree enables them to be properly handled.

It is pleasant for stables to face south, and the use of south-facing hatches allows for this: (see Fig. 2.8, which shows an economical stable yard). In this yard, the horses all face south but are tended from a central open driveway. Labour is thus reduced to a minimum under a traditional system of management.

Location of both tack and feed rooms is important as they are central to stable routines. The siting of the barn and muck heap are also critical. There is a possible advantage in siting the muck heap down-hill, if the yard is on a slope, since an empty barrow is easier to push up an incline.

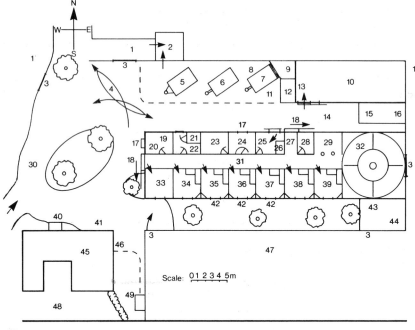

Key

1. Field
2. Field shelter/sick box
3. Gate
4. Lorry manoeuvring area
5. Caravan
6. Lorry or horse trailer
7. Trailer parked
8. Shavings
9. Platform
10. Barn for hay and shavings
11. Barrows
12. Ramp up
13. Tools
14. Delivery road
15. Tractor shed
16. Lean-to
17. Window
18. Sliding doors
19. Telephone
20. Office
21. WC
22. Changing
23. Tack room
24. Wash room
25. Feed room
26. Fire point
27. Exit
28. Dry room
29. Electric grooming bay
30. Drive
31. Passage for box access
    (N.B. hay and feed without
    entering stable)
32. Horse walker with roof
33. Wash and utility box
34. Box 1
35. Box 2
36. Box 3
37. Box 4
38. Box 5
39. Box 6
40. Front door
41. Car parking
42. Open hatchways, horses'
    lookout
43. Lean-to
44. Jump store
45. House
46. Back door
47. Manege 20 m × 60 m
48. Garden
49. Box gallery

Fig. 2.8 Example of a stable yard for six horses.

1. Select, pleasing locality, good site, tolerant neighbours, access to services, free-draining land and southerly aspect.

2. Access to training facilities to complement manege, etc. In particular, good safe hacking.

3. Aesthetically pleasing (looks good and appropriate to site and function), e.g. tiled roof towards house.

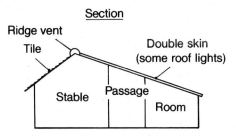

4. Labour-saving layout (see plan).

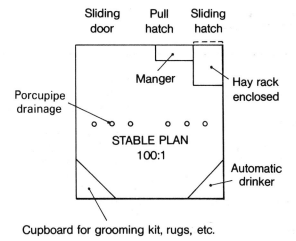

5. Labour-saving features particularly to help with routine stable duties, i.e. feeding hay and concentrates, watering, grooming, mucking out.

6. Design for safety and freedom from accidents.

7. Provide for fire fighting and emergency evacuation, e.g. hose reel in building handy to barn. Telephone. Two exits. Also, prevailing wind blows from house to stable to barn.

8. Design to minimize disease, e.g. low dust (hay barn downwind), good ventilation. Sick box.

9. Easy to clean and low maintenance.

10. Privacy for house occupants when off-duty.

Fig. 2.8 Cont'd. Features of the stable yard.

If muck is to be put into a skip or trailer for removal from the site, a sloping non-slip ramp will be required. The ramp should be sited so as to take advantage of any gradient and this could be a key factor in overall layout.

The major problem of feed rooms is that of rodents. Feed should be stored in metal bins. Sacks should be stored on low benching erected so as to allow for it to be swept under. A high degree of cleanliness and hygiene is essential: spilt food is best retrieved from difficult corners with a heavy-duty vacuum cleaner. Food is moved fastest with a round scoop, but there should be a set of trial scales so that a check can be kept on the weight of a scoop of different ingredients. If there is a barley or linseed boiler it should be sited beside a window to allow for the escape of steam.

There should be two distinct areas in the tack room – one for cleaned tack and the other (or dirty area) for working in. The dirty area should be equipped with a sink and draining board, with a source of both hot and cold water. There must also be a high saddle horse for cleaning saddles as well as a bridle hook. Provision must be made for dirty tack awaiting cleaning. The clean area should catch the eye when entering the room; there must be space for bandages, rugs, head collars, whips, lunge gear, etc. Metal trunks are rodent-proof and if set on strong board shelves provide neat storage for rugs out of season. The tack room should have a low-heat source to warm the air sufficiently to prevent condensation. The tack room should also have a source of heat for its human users; a minimum working temperature is a legal requirement. A fan heater will generally suffice. No reasonable employer minds heating a tack room, but anyone would object if the door is constantly open. Spring closures for doors keep the electricity bill down and make life easier for staff. A wall socket for a radio or cassette player will also be appreciated when tack is being cleaned. Radios should never be so loud that they disturb the atmosphere of the yard or that emergency instructions cannot be heard.

Provision for fire is essential but expensive; the local Fire Authority will be glad to give advice on the equipment needed, numbers of extinguishers, and so on. They are the experts and the Fire Prevention Officer's advice should be followed. He will visit the premises on request and his experienced eye may well detect dangers which can be eliminated by simple re-arrangement. In very small establishments, buckets containing sand are a cheap and easy provision for dealing with fire. Water buckets will also be needed and the best buckets for this purpose are those with round bottoms which cannot be used for anything else. They are hung up by the water trough ready for use. However, there should always be one or more fire extinguishers. There are various types of fire extinguisher;

those coloured blue contain powder which can be used to extinguish fires of all types and which is highly effective. Additionally, there should be a fire hose of sufficient length to reach all points on the premises. Fire hoses and other fire-fighting equipment should be checked or tested regularly; when testing a hose, it must be fully unwound before it operates at full force. Larger complexes will need a special fire hydrant point and additional equipment.

Doors might be locked when a fire breaks out, so a small axe should be available; strong bolt-cutters are needed in case a gate is padlocked or there is a stallion on a chain. Alarm systems can be simple or complicated: metal rotary fire gongs are not loud enough – an old school hand bell is far better. Larger establishments should have a small electric fire siren, and if it is likely there will be a large number of people around the premises, there should be several points from which the siren can be set off. Some yards may consider the installation of panic buttons to raise an alarm; these should not be exposed to accidental knocks and must be clearly signed.

In selecting building materials, the need to maintain a pleasant climate within the stable is paramount. A roof with good thermal properties will reduce rapid temperature changes. The worst type of roof is a low south-sloping one of galvanized iron; it results in excessive overheating on a pleasant summer's day and drips with condensation at night. A boarded roof covered with roofing felt works well and looks best if roofing felt tiles are used. Traditional tiles look good, but they need a strong supporting roof structure. Corrugated cement sheets – they no longer contain asbestos – are cheap but they need spraying on the underside with insulating material once they are set in place. Stables made of wood provide a pleasant environment for horses, but tend to get eaten. Ideally, they should have a smooth interior right up to the eaves, thus avoiding the problem. If only kicking boards are to be provided up to 1.2 m (4 ft) high, the area above the boards should be lined to stop the timber ribs being chewed.

The doorway is the second area of destruction by horses. Ideally, every wooden stable door should be fitted with an anti-weave grid to reduce chewing of the doorway. Anti-weave grids can be supplied by most manufacturers at no extra cost in lieu of a top door. Some wooden stables have the window beside the door; it is far better to specify that the window be set in the opposite wall. This lets in more light if not under an underhang and the window will not be obscured by the top door, if fitted. The window should be an opening one, protected by bars or mesh on the inside. The best forms of window ventilation are the 'Sheringham system' or louvres as both direct cold air upwards so that it mixes with the warm air in the stable. Louvres have the advantage of less intrusion into the stable and so are safer. Stables should have an opening in the ridge to allow warm stale air to escape.

Floors are a great problem. They should be non-slip, hard-wearing and should not strike cold; provision must be made for drainage. The cheapest floor is one of rammed chalk which works well on well-drained soils but needs maintenance. Porous tarmac laid on a bed of stones also works well, but drainage can be a problem. Drains within stables tend to harbour disease and are difficult to clear if blocked. The exception is a properly installed system of 'porcupipes' which provide a row of small holes across the floor. Concrete is the most commonly used flooring material and is sometimes laid without a drainage slope because bedding can absorb the urine. Generally, it is better laid with falls to a back corner outlet and so into an open drain channel. This is easy to keep clean and will not harbour vermin. Overall design unity, ease of work and personal preferences must all be taken into account.

Facilities

Labour must be used more effectively as it becomes more expensive. Most stables require that many hours be spent in steady work such as keeping stabled brood mares fit, getting horses up from grass, routine exercise of fit horses, and limbering-up or cooling off after schooling or other strenuous work. This is very labour-intensive, and much of the steady work can be done on the horse-walker. While four horses are exercising on the walker, their boxes can be mucked out. The early horse-walkers tended to pull the horse's head up unless side-reins were used. The popular modern designs allow the horse to be free in a moving pen between the inner and outer rails. If the horse-walker is outdoors, the walkway must receive particular care: sand and shavings over concrete seems to provide the best service.

Military stables used to include lunge rings and these are still provided in some racing yards. Indoor schools tend to be costly. Generally, lungeing can be done in an arena which also provides for riding. For working horses, an outdoor arena measuring 20×60 m is ideal; a little extra width is helpful if it is proposed to put a show jumping course on it. A useful compromise is an outdoor arena or school together with a 20 m^2 barn which allows for work in bad weather and is also useful for breaking.

The floor material of arenas is a controversial subject. Indoors, the traditional mixture is sand and wood shavings or sawdust, together with salt or fullers' earth to retain moisture. Outdoors, water is the main problem. Good drainage is essential, and this means that the drains must

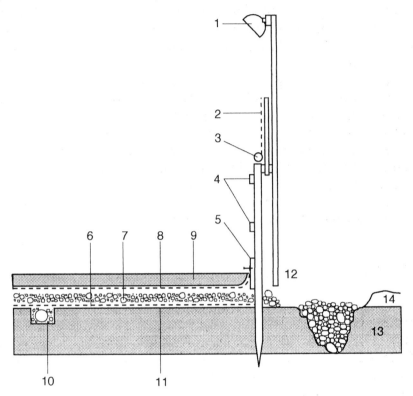

Key
1. Lights as high as practicable
2. Sight screen to 2 m where necessary
3. Irrigation system
4. At least 1.3 m high surround rails on inside of posts
5. Treated timber edge boards
6. Permeable membrane to stop stones sinking into the earth
7. Layer of stone for firm base and drainage
8. Second permeable membrane to stop stones rising
9. Riding surface
10. Drains as necessary (above ground arenas surrounded by French drains may not need drains below the riding surface)
11. Ground surface levelled
12. Riding surface must be above normal ground level to help drainage
13. 'French' or 'catchwater' drain
14. Topsoil removed and site levelled

Fig. 2.9 Construction of an outdoor arena. (Surface: sand, wood or other products.)

be laid, covered with stones laid on a membrane so they do not sink into the soil and topped with a second membrane to prevent the stones coming upwards, and a topping of the chosen surface material. In essence, the process is to build upwards from ground level away from the water table. This is shown in Fig. 2.9. Sand is still favoured as a surface because it does not degrade, but it can ride deep. This problem can be solved by the choice of sand or adding in elements to provide a firmer footing. The weekly and hourly amount of maintenance required is a further consideration. (An excellent but inexpensive booklet on the construction of all-weather riding arenas is available from the British Horse Society.)

A cantering track can be made cheaply by having the topsoil scooped off and backfilling the excavation with about 10 cm (4 in) of sand. Drainage pipes may need to be fitted in low-lying spots. Such a track will not be 'all weather', nor will it be as good as a racing gallop, but a 2 furlong (400 m) track is very useful in terms of faster fitness. Cross country fences need not be big for training; they should provide a variety of possibilities and are best set out like a show jumping course. The fences will be best if take-offs and landings are kept topped up with sand so that they do not get deep in wet weather.

When an indoor school is to be built, its basic design will be similar to an agricultural barn with outward sloping kicking boards rising to a height of at least 1.35 m (4ft 6in) sloping outwards at 10°. A height of 4.3 m (14 ft) to the eaves is adequate. Wide doors are required both for deliveries and maintenance. Lighting is by clear panels for daytime, with strip lighting for evening use. (A booklet on lighting sports areas is available from the Chartered Institution of Building Services Engineers, Delta House, 222 Balham High Road, London SW12 9BS.) An ingenious arrangement to ensure that clients hiring schools in the evening pay for the electricity they use is to install a coin-operated meter and, as a warning signal, a flashing beacon which comes on minutes before the power cuts off to leave only safety lighting. There should be a viewing gallery, however small; it may normally only house the trainer or instructor, but should always allow for other spectators. The gallery should be well insulated and efficiently heated; indoor schools can be very cold places. A layout for an indoor arena is shown in Fig. 2.10.

Under the Fire Safety Regulations and Safety of Places of Sport Act 1987 there are measures to enforce safety standards at indoor sporting events for spectators. A licence will be needed where the sports entertainment is the principal purpose for which the premises are being used. Thus every riding school which intends putting on shows and has a public gallery should have a licence. Certainly a licence would be needed

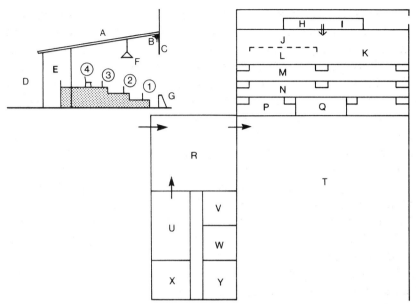

Key

A. Double skin roof
B. Loudspeaker
C. Heat retaining board
D. Section through the gallery
E. Passage
F. Halogen radiant heat lamp
G. Arena
H. Ramp
I. Steps
J. Standing
K. Gallery, space for wheelchairs
L. Row four

M. Row three
N. Row two
P. Row one
Q. Box for VIPs or dressage judge
R. Covered collecting area
T. Arena
U. Jump store
V. Competitors' viewing
W. Show office
X. Workshop
Y. Judges' box (show jumping)

Fig. 2.10 Layout of an indoor arena suitable for local shows.

if the public were to be charged for admission or were present in large numbers. Local authority safety experts will have to inspect the premises before a licence can be obtained.

Unless a side gallery is within the span of the building, the uprights (stanchions) would obscure the spectators' view, so an end gallery may be preferred. This is generally the less expensive option.

Accommodation

Accommodation for staff is often overlooked. In small establishments staff may live *en famille*, but a bigger enterprise may require purpose-built or converted accommodation. All too often this is scruffy and well-nigh uninhabitable. Good staff deserve good working and living conditions. In some cases, provision must be made for accommodating clients as well. All accommodation should be well maintained.

Essential requirements are a large boot park and area for wet-weather clothing – near to the back door. Drying areas for wet clothing are a must. Showers may suffice but hair dryers need plugs! Individual rooms are needed for all, except young clients who enjoy dormitory accommodation. Rooms must be able to cope with riding boots and other equipment, including the occasional saddle. Wholesome food and plenty of it is also essential. In self-catering establishments the microwave oven has done wonders for the communal kitchen. (Any form of catering facility, however, must comply with the Food and Hygiene Act.) Caring for horses may not be highly remunerated and may entail long hours; it certainly deserves comfortable surroundings, warm and dry accommodation with adequate facilities and good food; the same measure of personal privacy and security is essential. There is no doubt that staff and clients who are disgruntled by their living conditions will create an unpleasant atmosphere and everyone will suffer.

3 Staff

Introduction

Competent and happy staff are crucial to the success of any business operation. The greatest care is needed in the recruitment and training of staff and all employees deserve a career structure which is in line with other industries. Satisfactory pay and conditions and a happy working atmosphere and environment are essential if people are to give of their best. Each member of staff is an essential link in the chain. Wise employers help their employees to appreciate that they are part of a team and the most important people in the industry.

Recruitment

Losing a member of staff does not necessarily mean immediate replacement by someone with similar skills. A job vacancy gives the employer an opportunity to review the position and to appraise the overall staff situation. It is the right moment to consider the total skills of the whole workforce as well as the present and future needs of the business. In some cases, of course, a person with identical skills may be essential – though no two people are alike in personal attributes. In most cases, though, the employer should consider not only the skills that have been lost because an employee has moved on, but also the skills which will be needed in the future. This is as important in a small establishment as it is in a larger one. The key lies in finding the right person for the particular job. The terms and conditions of the job are also important. Working with horses may be a vocation, but 'job satisfaction' cannot compensate for meagre rewards!

Job specification

It is essential to have a job specification. Before advertising for a new recruit, the employer should write out a full description of the job and what it entails, along with the characteristics of the ideal candidate. These will range from training, qualifications and experience, to personal qualities and attitudes. It may well be that the 'ideal candidate' does not exist, and so it is necessary to list the various characteristics sought as either 'essential' or 'desirable'.

Adaptability is an important asset in the horse industry: some people can learn new skills very quickly, but all horse staff must be adaptable. A candidate may lack a required skill and yet be so good in all other respects that they rapidly become a key member of the team. In general, an enthusiastic attitude is more important than minor technical shortcomings. Training and education can provide the required skill and knowledge. They have an essential part to play at all staffing levels. Staff selection and training are inter-related. An existing employee may deserve promotion and yet need more training in a skill essential to the job. In such a case it may be worth deferring the appointment until the person is ready.

Listing the desirable characteristics of a proposed employee is not difficult. A checklist might be:

- *Age and physical factors*
Minimum and maximum ages. Health. Physique. Bearing. Speech. First impressions – these are of importance in a receptionist, for example. Ability to cope with pressure and stress is something not to be overlooked.
- *Attainments*
Education – general and special. Qualifications and experience. Past training. Training potential. Special knowledge and skills.
- *Aptitudes and interests*
Good with figures? Likes problem-horses? Development and implementation of new ideas.
- *Disposition*
Suitable for the job? Gregarious or solitary personality? Own initiative or routine?
- *Background*
Personal lifestyle and habits. (Family commitments can affect holidays and overtime.) Religious observances. Such restrictions are acceptable but should be known at the outset. The horse industry is demanding of people's time. If accommodation is offered, how will the applicant adjust away from home?

● *Career plans*

How the applicant sees the job is important. A career structure is important to those who wish to train to work with horses. Ambitions and potential must be considered. What are the job prospects? Promises that cannot be met should not be made.

Once the 'ideal candidate' is identified on paper, the vacancy can be advertised. Advertising may be internal, in local newspapers, and in the national equestrian press. Job vacancies should also be notified to the Department of Employment and to students through the various county colleges of agriculture with equestrian departments.

Recruitment agencies are becoming more prominent in the equestrian sector. For a small fee they provide a confidential service for employers and employees. Confidentiality is an important consideration for both parties and the use of Box Numbers in advertising can be useful.

Drafting advertisements is an art. The advertisement should outline the job, make it appear attractive, and invite those interested to send for further details, whether by letter or telephone. The employer should prepare an information sheet which includes a detailed job specification and sets out the wages and other conditions, such as accommodation, keep of own horse, time off, transport, etc. This sheet should be sent to each enquirer. Telephone inquiries should be answered immediately: the pre-prepared information sheet can be slipped straight into an envelope and put in the post. In larger establishments, an application form may be desirable; in every case applicants should be asked to produce a brief career outline or curriculum vitae and a letter of application. This should set out a personal resumé as well as the applicant's qualifications and experience. It should also say why the applicant is looking for a new job and when available to start. Employers should ask for one or two referees who can vouch for the candidate's character, abilities and experience. It should be made clear to candidates that references will always be checked.

Once the information is to hand, a preliminary selection can be made. Filling any job vacancy should be regarded as an important task. If there are few applicants it may be best to see them all on an informal basis until the appointment is made. Many positions are filled successfully in this way.

More senior jobs may attract many potentially suitable applicants and more formal procedures are needed. A short-list of six or so people should be made, and a day set aside for the interviews. Candidates should be invited for the morning which can be spent showing them round the premises, introducing them to other staff (if any) and chatting informally, answering questions as they arise. Lunch may be taken buffet-style, and formal interviews follow. Often by the end of lunch the interviewer has a fair idea of who the best candidate is – assuming that the candidate still shows interest in the job! But the interviewer should keep an open mind; first impressions are not necessarily the best ones.

Interviewing

Interviews are of many types, but job selection, annual appraisal and disciplinary interviews are the most important. Everyone in business needs to grasp the basic techniques, most of which are common to all interviews. Both interviewer and interviewee must be properly prepared, and this is one reason why preparation of an adequate job specification is so important. The person conducting the interview must have studied the relevant information in advance.

Interviews should be planned, but a large desk and very formal setting are not necessarily advantageous. An annual appraisal interview for each member of staff is ideally informal as its purpose is to discuss the individual's progress, job perceptions and career development. Comfortable chairs and informality will be the order of the day. Disciplinary interviews warrant different considerations and should be more formal.

Selection interviews require special techniques as both parties need to get to know one another. The first few minutes should be spent putting the interviewee at ease and adjusting lines of communication. Rapport must be established. Someone who is tense may have difficulty in marshalling their thoughts and not say what they intended to say. The interviewee should be told the proposed format for the interview and be encouraged to ask questions.

At a selection interview the following points should be covered:

- The duties of the job.
- Duration of employment. Is the appointment a permanent one or is it seasonal or temporary?
- The working hours and time-off.
- The wage offered and how it is paid – weekly or monthly and whether in cash or by cheque.
- Overtime. Hourly rate of pay or whether time-off in lieu is given. Extra payments for work away from base, e.g. a groom travelling with a horse to a show, should be settled.

- Other conditions. Board and lodging, keep of own horse, use of car, entry in competitions, etc. If the post is residential, the standard of accommodation offered should be discussed, the interviewee having already seen it.
- The person to whom the employee is responsible and what other staff are to be the employee's superiors.

Skilled interviewers use questions as a means of going forward and always remain in control of the situation. Questions asked should not prompt 'yes' or 'no' answers. Rudyard Kipling's words give the clue to the correct approach:

'I keep six honest serving men,
    They've taught me all I know.
Their names are "What" and "Why" and "When",
    And "How" and "Where" and "Who".'

Kipling-type questions invite the person being interviewed to open out, and avoid one word answers. Other good lines of approach are:

'Tell me about ...'
'Yes, go on.'
'Why do you say that?'
'Do you prefer ...?'
'So you feel upset about ... Why?'
'So what you are saying is ...'

In this way, the interviewer listens and understands; from time to time the interviewer should check to see that what has been said is correctly understood. Some answers at interviews are too long and wordy – whether because of nervousness or verbosity. A firm 'Right, thank you' may help to stop the flow and take matters on to the next point.

Once the candidates have been interviewed, and providing references have already been taken up, a decision can be made. In the horse industry, it is seldom necessary to delay making an appointment. The selected candidate should be invited back to the interview room and offered the job. Once the offer has been accepted, the disappointed applicants can be thanked and sent on their way.

Notes are a useful aid to concentration during any interview but can be overdone. Only outline notes need be taken during a selection interview. The position is different at a disciplinary or annual appraisal interview. In those cases, careful notes should be made and put on record for future reference.

Employment and employing staff

Whether someone working on the premises is an employee in the legal sense is not an academic question. Employees are those who have entered into or who work under a contract of employment. (Contracts of employment are discussed in Chapter 5.) It is a legal requirement that workers working at least eight hours a week are given a written statement of the terms of their employment within two months of starting work. They must also be covered by employers' liability insurance in case they are injured or contract certain diseases whilst carrying out their job. Employees also fall under the scope of the National Insurance scheme. Casual helpers – such as the schoolgirl who lends a hand at weekends – are not usually classified as employees. However, if such a volunteer is kicked, she may be entitled to claim compensation from the business if the injury resulted from negligence. It is not possible to contract out of liability for negligence which results in death or personal injury, even if an indemnity has been signed by the the casual helper and her parents. This is a result of the Unfair Contract Terms Act 1977, of which s. 2 (1) provides that it is not possible to exclude or restrict liability in negligence for personal injury or death 'by reference to any contract term or to a notice given to persons generally or to particular persons'.

Employees tend to take their example from the person immediately above them. A cheerful and hard working Head Lad or Head Girl with high standards normally means that there is an excellent atmosphere in the yard. However, even a person of that calibre will get depressed if the employer is morose, weighed down with problems or acts irrationally. Employers should always be fair, predictable and reasonable. The atmosphere in the yard is important for the horses as well; human feelings and tensions communicate themselves to horses. If the horses are relaxed and happy they can use their energies to best advantage; sullen horses do not thrive or perform well.

Staff are usually the most expensive business cost and it is essential to the success of any business that staff have the right attitudes and skills. If one discounts the cost of the premises, labour costs usually amount to some 60 per cent of the total cost of keeping a horse. If this percentage is to be reduced, either the staff must be paid less – in which case they are probably of little use – or they should be able to look after more horses. This does not mean that staff should be overworked or that the horses' care should be skimped. It means that labour should be used more efficiently.

This requires labour-saving equipment as well as good routines. In some yards, the care of horses needs as much labour nowadays as it did centuries ago, but in almost every other area of activity, progress has meant better and more efficient use of human resources. Only pack animals can be exercised as such, and only polo grooms can ride one horse while leading four others. Even they need assistance to get out of the yard, and the practice can be hazardous.

Traditionally, hunters were exercised on the basis of one being ridden and the other led, and in many cases they still are. Today, horse-walkers, equine swimming pools and treadmills offer possibilities for exercise which require less labour. Routine stable tasks also offer scope for greater efficiency.

In considering the employment of staff and the labour needed, the review should also include consideration of whether it is better to invest the money in a piece of equipment or another pair of hands. The matter should be costed carefully. Many of the more successful equine businesses are very well equipped, although it is debatable whether the good equipment has bred success or vice versa. Success certainly attracts high calibre staff and in this sense 'success breeds success.' Success in business often starts with the selection of the right staff.

Motivation

Most people are motivated to work by a mixture of pride and profit (Fig. 3.1). Pride is an innate human characteristic, just like the instincts of hunger and self-protection. It is pride which impels a homemaker to keep the house neat and tidy, and pride makes employees ambitious and successful.

In today's world, an individual's needs are greater because one's expectations are higher. Advertising and the consumer society make almost everyone feel that they 'need' items which were considered as luxuries only a generation ago. There is also the increased reliance on the use of credit facilities to buy things immediately rather than on saving for something specific. Financial benefits and rewards therefore loom large when someone is considering whether to take a job, although so-called 'fringe benefits' are also important, as discussed later.

The most valuable resource of any organization is its human assets – the employees. The manager – the person in day-to-day charge – is the most crucial staff member. All too often the typical manager is merely average. A successful business needs a successful and well-motivated manager who is a leader, motivator, team builder, listener, good

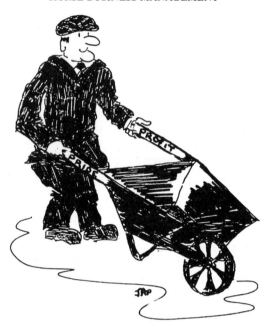

Fig. 3.1 People are like wheelbarrows – to make them go forward you must apply pressure to both handles – *pride* and *profit*.

communicator and able to delegate successfully . The good manager always looks to the future and plans efficiently. He/she is not afraid to make decisions and has the right priorities. Good managers gain in self-confidence because they are trusted. In turn, they trust others and, having established good routines, leave others to put them into practice. In this way they have the time necessary to concentrate on those matters which call for their own expert judgement and decision.

The good employer will pay staff the best and most competitive rates he/she can afford. The good employer will ensure that each member of staff feels secure in the job, enjoys good living conditions and a satisfactory and pleasant working environment. He/she will also ensure that they work in such a way that they are stretched and fulfilled. Most people respond well to trust, challenge and recognition as well as to financial reward. Staff should feel secure and part of the enterprise. They should be consulted and respected. Good work should be praised; less satisfactory work should be queried. Management mistakes should be honestly admitted. 'Please', 'thank you' and 'we' are words which are crucial for success. Some wit in industry produced 'rules' for stifling initiative: the rules in Fig. 3.2 are based on them.

1. Regard any new idea from the staff with suspicion – because it's new and because it's from below.
2. Insist that staff who want to use their initiative present their proposals in writing, in duplicate.
3. Ask staff to challenge and criticize each other's proposals (this saves the task of deciding – just pick any survivors).
4. Withhold praise and express criticism freely; this keeps staff on their toes and makes them feel vulnerable, so stops them getting too cocky.
5. Treat identification of problems as a sign of failure; this discourages people from letting you know when some areas are not going smoothly.
6. Keep total control and make sure that anything which can be counted is counted frequently.
7. Make decisions to reorganize or change policies in secret and then spring them on people unexpectedly – they may admire your decisiveness.
8. Ensure that any request for information is fully justified in writing – you don't want your business secrets falling into the wrong hands.
9. Delegate to the Head Lad, Head Girl or your Assistant responsibility for implementing any unpopular decisions you have made.
10. Above all else never forget that you already know all that you need to know about this business.

Fig. 3.2 The blasé manager's recipe for success (and stifling initiative).

Remuneration

Remuneration is a synonym for reward and is not merely proper wages. It includes all the benefits attached to a job such as board and lodging, keep of own horse, use of vehicle and so on. Accommodation provided for staff must be dry and warm in winter, and the cost of the necessary heating is inevitably expensive. Some staff accommodation in the industry uses metered heating for which the employees are expected to pay on an 'as used' basis. In some cases meters are unfairly and improperly set so that the staff pay over and above the true cost. In general staff who understand and feel a part of the business will not waste money and with encouragement will often find ways of saving it.

It may be practicable and in some cases essential to provide meals for staff. Where young staff are employed and provided with accommodation, nutritious and regular meals are essential.

If staff are allowed to keep their own horses, the costing is more complicated. There is the cost of keeping the horse, the loss of potential profit on another horse that might have been stabled and the cost of the time the employee spends in looking after the horse. Another perquisite may be the use of a vehicle in free time. Free use of a washing machine may be another benefit.

Training is often part of the package in the non-thoroughbred world especially where someone is progressing through examinations. Agreements ought to be set down in writing so that both parties can see the total value of the package and assess its implications.

Staff training

Staff development is an important aspect of management. It takes two forms:

- In-house training, which utilizes the skills within the business to train staff.
- External or agency training. This may take a variety of forms – day release courses, short courses, study days, attendance at conferences and so on.

Training is recognized as a sound investment today, and there should be a clear agreement as to the training programme. Young staff will often be ambitious to progress to jobs of greater responsibility which demand new skills. If they are provided with adequate training they will be content and not anxious to move on quickly. The various factors affecting the acquisition of a skill are set out in Table 3.1.

Table 3.1 Factors affecting skill acquisition.

External	Teacher	Student
Environment	Enthusiasm	Physical ability
Facilities	Empathy	Age
Distractions	Skill at subject	Sex
Time available	Skill as teacher	Maturity
	Skill as motivator	Intelligence
		State of mind
		Motivation
		Enthusiasm
		Time
		Money
		Preconceptions
	Duration and frequency of practice	

In general it is desirable that all employees end the day feeling that they have learned something.

Skill has been described as competence built on knowledge and understanding. Attainment of skill in this wider sense is not just the capacity to perform a particular task, nor is it the empty acquisition of factual knowledge. It is the coming together of competence, knowledge and understanding and as such it is a proper goal for both educators and trainers.

Because, to make the best progress, it is necessary to gain both education and training, many school leavers intent on a horse career plan to go to college (Fig. 3.3). Many of the specialist college horse courses are eligible for discretionary grant aid.

There are many new and developing techniques which can be utilized cost-effectively for staff training. The use of them means that it is cheaper to train existing staff than to rely on outside consultants or advisers.

Training needs are partly exposed by staff appraisal interviews, which should be held for each employee annually. The purpose of such appraisals is to discuss the person's hopes, aspirations, progress and training needs. The training needs of new employees should be discussed and agreed at the initial selection interview. What is agreed then should form part of the terms of the contract of employment. Another set of

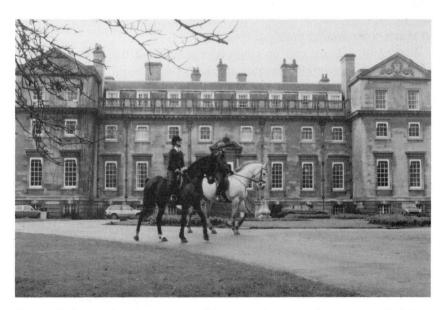

Fig. 3.3 College students have a wonderful opportunity to start their careers with the best of preparation.

needs can be identified by considering the objectives of the business and analysing the skills necessary to meet them. Checking the existing skills of the present staff will identify any new skills likely to be required.

Student-centred learning

There are fashions and in-terms in all branches of management; 'student-centred learning' is in this category but is a convenient shorthand for an important concept. The term emphasizes that teaching is about students and not about teachers and that the correct criterion in training is the amount that is learned rather than what is taught. The name also describes the technique. Students learn by doing, feeling, experiencing and enquiring. 'I hear and I forget; I see and I remember; I do and, only then, I understand.'

Students should be encouraged to learn from every small daily occurrence and not only from formally taught sessions. Simulation exercises are important and just as senior managers attend expensive courses where they play 'management games' and then discuss and analyse their approach to fictional problems, simulation can be utilized in all areas. For example, the plaiting of manes and tails can be learnt first on model necks and docks using bale string instead of hair. Leadership skills can be tested using jump poles, oil drums and ropes to perform a specific task, such as crossing a river without getting a load wet – just as in military leadership practical tests.

Riding instruction can be given on the basis of the student-centred technique. For example, instead of instructing a pupil 'Raise your left hand', the instructor might say 'Look where your left hand is now and consider how the horse is going, then try your hand a little higher and a little lower and see if it makes a difference'. In this way, the students learn to cope on their own and become aware of the relationship between rider and horse.

Teaching using this technique may seem more difficult at first. For example, the old routine of riding in formation may be easier, but better learning and teaching results from a compromise. Junior and novice riders at a riding school might first ride in formation, but then be allowed to ride in open order to try out the newly-acquired skills.

The process of learning

A skill is ability in a task, especially one acquired by training. It is usually made up of several smaller skills. Thus, when driving a car, to change gear requires clutch and accelerator operation, followed by gear change and then clutch and accelerator adjustment in opposite sequence, all performed without looking. This skill can be broken down into separate parts: e.g. learning the position of each gear first by looking and changing gear, learning to dip the clutch and let it up again smoothly without changing gear. The same analysis can be applied to any skill acquired by training.

The sequence of teaching a skill is:

- The complete skill is demonstrated at normal speed in context.
- The complete skill is then demonstrated very slowly so that each part can be identified.
- Each component skill is demonstrated and exactly what is involved is analysed.
- The student learns each of the component parts.
- The student then puts them together into the complete skill.
- The skill is practised to achieve satisfactory speed, efficiency, fluency and competence.

This can be summarized as 'I do it normally, I do it slow. You do it with me, now off you go.'

Students can learn because the instructor advises on every detail or by making their own mistakes. 'Feedback' is important in teaching, whether it is external – from the teacher – or intrinsic – from the student who recognizes that the horse did not respond as required. Riding instructors who encourage intrinsic feedback develop riders with 'feel'.

Table 3.2 illustrates some activities that enable students to learn more about horses; not all of them are obvious.

Examinations

Good training requires 'markers' to show achievement; training for dressage enables both horse and rider to tackle more demanding tasks. For most skills, the 'markers' will be a series of graduated examinations or tests. There are in fact over 70 examinations in the British horse world, and no employer can be aware of the significance of each one. The development of National Vocational Qualifications (NVQs) has helped to promote a national system.

Continuous assessment is an important aspect of modern examinations. The system relies on the candidate's trainer to chart the individual's progress. In this way, each aspect of learning is checked rather than the small random sample of the traditional practical examination. It is

Table 3.2 Enabling activities. Activities that ENABLE students to learn more about horses.

ACTIVE			PASSIVE	
The student does			The student has done to him/her	
Creating	Solving	Using	Indirect[1]	Direct[2]
Write an essay, paper, notes or a book.	An objective test (test of facts)	The student will use his/her knowledge	Read a book, magazine, paper, map, wallchart or poster	A study or tour visit
Produce a project	Practical test of problem solving	Practical practice (common in riding schools)	Watch and listen to film, video, tape, slides, television	A demonstration
Give a talk	Experiment to solve a problem	Role play	Listen to radio, tape, record	A led discussion
Make a model	Knowledge test	Discussion groups	Smell various odours	Instructor answers questions
Draw a picture, plan or diagram	Comprehension test	Business games	Feel shape and texture of various objects	Dictated or copied notes
Take a photograph	Application test	Practical competition	Visit show; study trade stands	External reinforcement (by the instructor)
Make a film, video, tape, slides	Buzz group (impromptu discussion on a specific topic)	Practical examination of competence	Visit sales competition, display demonstration, exhibition	External motivation (by the instructor)
Act	Judge a competition	Teaching machines audio and/or visual	Study hand-outs, selected passages from books and other publications and papers	A lecture
Write a short story that is well researched	Place in order of merit	Programmed learning	Enter an environment which is an experience in itself, e.g. The Spanish Riding School in Vienna	
Any form of synthesis where something is built up or put together.	Identification test	Fill in hand-out	Be frightened by an experience	
	Answer questions	Use teaching pack	Enjoy an experience	
	Literary search	Demonstrate skill		
	Evaluate information			

[1] May be instructor guided
[2] Instructor based activities

sometimes alleged against this system that instructors will be biased in favour of their own trainees, but a moment's reflection shows that this is not so, since passing someone who is not 'up to standard' merely reflects on the instructor's reputation.

In practice, continuous assessment is well proven in other industries, and is often linked to a final traditional examination with an appropriate weighting. In some examinations series, external moderators or verifiers are used to make random checks to ensure that the system has been fairly and properly applied. With experienced moderators or verifiers, this system gives more accurate results than conventional examinations; it is also far more cost-effective! A similar system under NVQs allows approved yard managers to assess their trainees on the practical units of the examination and these results to be subject to random tests by verifiers.

Multiple-choice examination questions provide another accurate and cost-effective scheme. The entire syllabus can be swiftly checked; there are no personality or examination nerves problems, and misinterpretation of the questions is avoided. (Such questions need rigorous testing before use.)

Examining is an imperfect science, but it should at least be seen to be fair, reasonable, and to produce graduates with a thorough understanding.

Supervision

The key person in the team is the Head Lad, Head Girl, stud groom or supervisor; the title used is unimportant, but the person's role is vital. He or she is both team leader and taskmaster. The supervisor sets the standards required, whether of cheerfulness, time-keeping, loyalty, hard work, smartness, attention to detail or anything else. The team leader's personality must be buoyant so that morale can be maintained at difficult times. Different yards have different expectations of both supervisor and other staff, but a suggested division of responsibilities between supervisor and other staff members is shown in diagrammatic form in Table 3.3.

Table 3.3 Division of responsibilities between the Head Lad/Girl and other staff.

Supervisor	Staff
Requirement A competent worker able not only to do the skills but also to teach, supervise and organize them. Able to assist and deputize for the manager.	*Requirement* A competent worker who is skilful and proficient within the range of routine tasks.
Qualities and abilities Confident, reliable, inspires confidence, gives orders without offence, maintains discipline and high standards, keeps accurate records, encourages and gives training to junior staff. Identifies with the aims and objectives of the establishment. Discreet and loyal. Safe. Leads by example.	*Qualities and abilities* Works safely with thought, care and efficiency to an agreed plan.
Typical tasks Work organization. Horse care. Training and fitness to agreed plan. Care of facilities. Grassland practical management. Linking records with office use. Stud work to an agreed plan. Stable allocation	*Typical tasks* Stable routines. Basic horse handling. Feeding and watering. Routine health care. Riding to an agreed plan. Transporting. Keeping records. Grooming and stabled-horse care. Tractor driving tasks. Tack care.

Giving instructions

The supervisor must give instructions concerning the work to be done, but a mere instruction is often insufficient. In many cases it is appropriate not only to tell people what has to be done, but also to show them how to do it. This is especially so with newcomers and it is important for the supervisor to explain why the job should be done in that way and in some cases why the job is necessary at all! Understanding the importance of a job leads to pride in the work done. The supervisor should emphasize the important aspects of the task, especially safety.

Routines

Routines are a regular method of procedure, and since much work with horses is unvarying it is important that staff establish and follow good routines. This important subject is discussed further in Chapter 7 where suggested timetables are given. One reason for good routine is that horses are creatures of habit; routine makes them feel happy and secure and so they thrive and perform better. Horses can also be dangerous, and all good routines require that tasks are done in the safest possible way, thus minimizing or avoiding accidents. Many stable tasks are repetitive and following the agreed routine will be the most efficient way of doing the job. Effort is saved, productivity is increased, and high standards can be maintained.

The routine for keeping records, for example, ensures that accurate and up-to-date figures are available to provide management with the information needed to run the business efficiently. Good routine ensures that there is a daily programme, a place for everything and a check-list to ensure that all the chores are completed. In this way, the supervisor can, with a minimum of effort, run an efficient yard which is a pleasure to work in.

Safety

It is the responsibility of both employers and employees to ensure that safe working conditions are observed. The Health and Safety at Work Act 1974 imposes obligations upon both employers and employees to take reasonable care both of themselves and others, and people at work must not be exposed to unnecessary risks to their health or safety. Employers are obliged to provide a safe and healthy working environment: safe equipment, safe premises and safe systems of work.

The enforcement of the 1974 Act is in the hands of the local authority which inspects equestrian premises and advises upon compliance with the legislation. It is impossible to make any working premises absolutely safe and the employer's obligation is to ensure the health and safety of employees 'so far as is reasonably practicable'. A basic duty is also imposed upon all employees while at work, namely to act in the course of their employment with reasonable care for the health and safety of themselves, other workers and the general public, and to co-operate with the employer and anyone else upon whom a statutory duty or requirement is imposed, e.g. an inspector, to see that the relevant statutory provisions are observed. The effect of all this is that at any equine establishment all who work there, whether employees or otherwise, together with visitors, all come under the Act.

Buildings and all work places must be safe in construction and properly maintained. Safe equipment must be provided and properly maintained. Veterinary products and disinfectants must be safely stored and used. Gas bottles need special safe storage and appliances need professional installation and proper maintenance.

Where five or more people are employed, s. 2(3) of the Act obliges the employer:

'To prepare and, as often as may be appropriate, to revise a written statement of his general policy with respect to the health and safety at work of his employees, and the organization and arrangements for the time being in force for carrying out that policy, and to bring the statement and revision of it, to the notice of all his employees.'

Shorn of the legal verbiage, compliance with this requirement includes three elements: (a) a written safety policy, (b) organization, and (c) arrangements for carrying it out.

A written safety policy

Employers must prepare and issue a written policy statement outlining their health and safety philosophies. This must indicate the commitment of management and employees to the implementation of that policy. It need not be a lengthy document and the Health and Safety Executive have published a booklet *Writing Your Health and Safety Policy Statement* which is available from HMSO (ISBN 0 11885510 7) which gives guidance on preparing the statement and lays down the important points using page by page examples. The statement must cover the intent to comply with the statutory provisions and must lay particular emphasis on safe work routines and stress the importance of co-operation from the workforce and of good communications. It should be signed by the employer or a partner or senior director. The policy must be kept under review and the written statement amended when necessary.

Organization

Even in a small business it is necessary to have a clearly drawn picture of the line and functional responsibilities of the people responsible for health and safety. If necessary the statement should define the responsibilities of named senior and junior members of staff both with regard to health and safety generally and to emergency situations. Those named must have adequate information and authority to perform their responsibilities.

Arrangements

The arrangements for carrying out the policy must be tabulated clearly, e.g. line responsibility for health and safety. Likely hazards must be identified and listed together with rules and practices for avoiding them. The arrangements for dealing with fire, injury and other emergencies must be spelled out. The arrangements for providing instruction, training and supervision must also be made clear.

All this is really common sense, and of course a written statement does not prevent accidents; the policy must be implemented. Table 3.4 sets out a typical safety code for an equine business; this should be distributed to all staff. It is not the written policy required by the Act; that has to be written by the management of each business, according to its needs.

Table 3.4 Typical safety code.

- Consideration of safety for people must override all others.

- Be mindful of the safety of persons, stock and equipment.

- Do not use faulty equipment – report it to. . . .

- Personal: Secure long hair, keep finger nails trimmed, keep jewellery to a safe minimum, wear suitable clothing and footwear for the work being done. Wear a hard hat to current BSI specifications, adequately secured at all times when mounting, dismounting and riding; also when breaking and assisting with stallions at service. Wear gloves when there is a risk to hands through sudden pulls on lead ropes or lunge lines.

- Riding out: Only those with specific authority to do so may ride on the roads. Keep to the left. Keep led horses on the left of the handler. Avoid pavements and mown grass by houses. No smoking. After sunset, lights and reflective clothing must be worn whether riding or leading. Take care when passing pedestrians; particularly go slowly if passing them on bridleways. Show courtesy to other road users. Thank all drivers – whether they slow down or not. Abide by the BHS publication *Ride and Drive Safely*. Inform on route and time of return before departing the yard.

- Around the yard: Know and be able to apply the fire drill. No smoking except in the designated rest area. Tether horses for mucking-out.

- Stud: Avoid leading mares or stallions past each other, especially during the stud season. Avoid scented soaps and perfumes when working with stallions.

A proper first-aid kit must be provided and maintained in good order. Staff should be encouraged to seek immunization against tetanus. An effective rodent control programme must be maintained. Staff must be provided with protective clothing where appropriate, e.g. hard hats, and advised on their correct fitting, condition and use. Employees' attention should be drawn to matters of personal hygiene such as the need to wash hands before eating so as to guard against Weil's disease which is spread by vermin contamination.

Those working in dusty conditions or handling hay or bedding rife with fungal spores must be provided with respiratory protection equipment. Workers must be instructed in safe working procedures and there should be a planned programme of training which should include an induction programme for newcomers. The use of unsafe or makeshift equipment must not be condoned and there must be adequate supervision to see that safe working practices are taught and then observed. Damaged fingers result from failure to wear protective gloves, damaged toes from failing to wear protective boots, and damaged backs from faulty lifting techniques.

All new employees and trainees, for example, should be shown and trained how to handle, lift and carry correctly, and should be regularly checked. Correct technique reduces the likelihood of damage to the back or rupture; it reduces fatigue and improves efficiency. Further information on health and safety is given in Appendix 1.

Discipline and grievances

Every business except a small employer should have a formal disciplinary procedure so that the employee can be treated fairly and in accordance with natural justice if he/she steps out of line.

There should also be a grievance procedure so that employees know what to do if they are dissatisfied. Ideally, grievances should not reach a formal stage because good communications mean that the manager or supervisor has already spotted that something is amiss and initiated a discreet inquiry into the problem. The difficulty may be of a personal nature, and friendly counselling may be received and appreciated. The problem may arise from a misunderstanding or from a personality clash; again, once the cause is identified, a solution can be found. There should be a strong team concept in the business and the working team should be given the opportunity to ask questions and to discuss issues.

Discipline is a skill calling for sensitivity, courage and good judgement. A person who has done wrong will usually accept a fair reprimand and go back to work in reasonably good humour. Occasionally, it may be appropriate to be tolerant or turn a blind-eye, e.g. someone who had sat up all night with a sick horse would be justifiably aggrieved if, next day, they received more than a gentle reminder for a lapse in routine.

If an employee does fall seriously out of line, then a clear verbal warning should be issued. The employee must know the nature of the fault alleged against him/her, and be given a fair opportunity to state his/her case. The employee is entitled to appeal to a level of management not previously involved in the matter.

If a verbal warning is given, it should be recorded in the employee's file. A subsequent lapse may merit a further verbal warning, which should also be recorded. Termination of employment is a last resort, and its legal and practical implications are discussed in Chapter 5.

Equal opportunities

Any business should have and practise an equal opportunities policy, for example:

- All concerned with the business should offer equal opportunities to all people.
- Policies, communications and actions should be free of discrimination in terms of race, gender, age, marital status, religion, background, political and private beliefs, sexual persuasion and disability except on grounds of safety.
- Harassment will not be tolerated.
- Where appropriate and within financial and safety constraints, provision will be made for those with disabilities.

This policy concentrates on the positive when considering new applicants and promotions; the positive being the person's ability to do the job well as an integral member of the team.

4   The office

Introduction

Every business enterprise needs an office where the inevitable clerical work can be done, records stored and visitors received. Office work is just as important as work in the yard, and good organization can reduce the 'chores' aspect to a minimum. An office is essential to the efficient and profitable running of any business. In a small horse business, the office may well be a room in the house or even part of a room. Even in a home-based business, an effort should be made to provide separate accommo-dation from the family living-space. The principles of office organization are identical whether the office is part of the working complex (as this chapter assumes) or a room in a house.

Organization

Since offices are communication centres they should be strategically placed to intercept visitors, receive mail, store records which are available to the yard if needed, and keep in touch with staff. In practical terms this means that ideally the office should be sited by the entrance gate and clearly labelled as 'Office and Reception' so as to leave no doubt that visitors should call there.

If possible, there should be a separate reception area. There should be a bell connected to a yard or house bell and a notice stating that if the office is unmanned, the visitor should ring and wait. Dependent on the arrangement of the office, a buzzer can be useful even if the office is staffed full-time. Even if there is a full-time secretary, arrangements should be made for other members of the staff to undertake reception duties if he or she is absent. A notice outside the reception door should show the hours of attendance and give a telephone number for emergency contact. The notice can show other useful information such as the nearest pay telephone, the owner's address, etc.

Some riding schools undoubtedly lose business because of the poor first impression created by the reception area and office. If it is poorly decorated, furnished badly and is dirty and disorganized, customers may reasonably assume that the remainder of the establishment is equally shoddy. It is not necessary to spend a great deal of money in order to give the right impression, but a neat and tidy layout and cleanliness must be the order of the day.

A stud farm or dealing yard must necessarily set similar first impressions. There must be a suitable area in which to make the bargain and deal with any necessary paperwork. A pound or two spent on refreshments for a customer in such cases will only be a tiny percentage of the overall transaction. The smaller business has neither the means to afford nor the need for a smart foyer with a receptionist and well-dressed sales-people eager to close a deal, but the horse world can learn from other areas where such things are justified. Certainly, the reception areas at some of the bigger studs warn potential customers that the prices are likely to be high. Some training yards have the rule that owners should visit by appointment only and this certainly makes sense. Where this rule applies, the yard has a drinks party for all owners once a month, thus establishing camaraderie between the owners who feel that they are members of a rather exclusive club. These trainers may well, on accountants' advice, be able to claim part of the costs of decorating and furnishing some rooms in their homes as a legitimate expense for tax purposes.

In many horse businesses the working office will be in the owner's house and the tack room will double as a reception area in the yard. Even here, attention should be paid to reception and office duties in the training of staff.

Office routines

For equestrian businesses, office routines can be divided into six main areas:

- people
- horses
- finance
- estate
- marketing
- competitions.

These subdivisions are very broad and not in any order of importance and the routines actually followed and records kept will depend on the nature of the enterprise.

People

Staff records must be maintained, not only to comply with legal requirements but for other purposes as well. There should be a personal file for each present and former employee and a general one for unsuccessful job applicants as well. Employees' personal files will include a copy of the written contract of employment, training programme, annual reviews, disciplinary notes, holidays and so on. PAYE and National Insurance records must also be maintained. Personal data kept in computerized form is now subject to control under the Data Protection Act 1987, which means that it must be made available to the individual on request as well as being securely guarded from intrusion. It also means that if personal records are kept on computer this fact should be notified and registered on a form from the post office. An Incident Book (formerly Accident Book) must be maintained in which any accidents can be recorded.

Horses

The records needed will depend on the nature of the enterprise; a stud will need different records from a riding school. There should be individual files for each horse giving purchase details, competition entries and performance, expenses, veterinary attention, farriery and any routine health treatment. Livery stables, studs and some other establishments need a monthly routine of invoicing and credit control. A useful system is to have separate books for veterinary routines and farriery which can be completed at the time of the visit. Carbon duplicate books are useful because the top copy can then be inserted in the individual horse's file while the duplicates remain in the yard. There should also be a Stock Book, Tack Book and possibly a Feed Book.

Finance

Accurate financial records are essential for legal, fiscal and control purposes. All expenses and income should be properly recorded in a form agreed with the accountant. Certain statutory PAYE and related records must be kept. General financial records should be prepared in a readily understandable way. Most equine business can use a single entry or cash analysis book, with the figures totalled monthly. In small businesses the record-keeper may well be the owner. In other cases, the secretary or person responsible for finance will be engaged on a part-time basis and use may be made of the local mobile farm secretarial service. However, even with professional help basic records must be kept on site – including a petty cash book. Any cash or other payments should be recorded as they come in and all cheques should be banked regularly. PAYE, income tax and National Insurance contributions are something not to be over-looked, and VAT records must be maintained and supporting documen-tation readily available in case of a visit from HM Customs and Excise who are not noted for their kind-heartedness or willingness to overlook errors and omissions.

Estate

This term covers the management of the land and buildings and any equipment and machinery, together with any associated agricultural or other enterprises. Again, the records can be kept simple but are important.

Marketing

Marketing strategy, advertising, public relations, new ideas and develop-ments, and monitoring marketing activities all need proper attention in the office. It is all too easy to be so involved in caring for the horses and the general routines of running the business that this area becomes neglected.

Competitions

Racing and competition stables need sound routines to cope with entries. In the racing world, not every entry made is followed up and this is an expensive feature of racing. Submitting entries may require the payment of subscriptions to various organizations, registration with a particular body and so on. Such matters all fall within this routine. Subscriptions to organizations should be paid as they fall due.

The keeping of records is a chore, especially when a conventional filing system is used. Staff will need strong motivation to keep records accurate and up-to-date. Only records which will be used should be kept; their usage will partly dictate the method of filing them. Records which are difficult in terms of access and retrieval mean that they will be used less and so are less worthwhile.

Equipment

The basic office equipment is a suitable desk and chair together with a filing cabinet. Second-hand office equipment is readily available, and little effort is required to produce a co-ordinated office image. Other essential equipment is a telephone, preferably with a fax and answering machine, a word processor (or typewriter) and a calculator (or a personal computer). The usual office supplies of notepaper, envelopes, carbon paper, paper clips and so on present no problem.

It may well be that most conventional office equipment is now obsolete in light of the ready availability of relatively cheap personal computers, although the time of the 'paperless office' is far off, and conventional records must necessarily be maintained.

Personal computers

Whether or not to purchase a computer – and if so which one – is a difficult question for many people. In fact, even a small business will benefit substantially. The costs of buying a small computer have tumbled over the last few years so that the outlay will not be major. However, deciding to buy a computer is not a simple matter. There are various models and each of them have different features.

The simplest type is a dedicated word processor which replaces the typewriter. This speeds up letter-writing and makes the handling of correspondence easy. It will also produce standard letters which can be 'personalized'. A standard letter can thus be sent to each client looking as if it has been personally typed, since the word processor will insert the individual's name and address and personal opening and a reference to the addressee's horse by name into a standard format.

Dedicated word processors can be very sophisticated but few of them are as powerful as personal computers.

Those in the horse business are well advised to purchase a personal computer since it will be more powerful and have more facilities than a simple word processor, if only because with a suitable program the computer can be used to do the accounts. It is not necessary to know how computers work in order to use them, though unfortunately the computer industry has created a jungle of jargon which is intensely annoying to those outside the specialist field. Computers become an obsession with some people, almost a religion; they insist on putting everything on computer and spend many happy hours playing with them. Much computerized information can be recorded more simply on paper and filed and be retrieved just as rapidly.

Independent computer consultants can advise on an appropriate system, but they mostly concentrate on the more sophisticated needs of complex businesses. Apart from specialist computer shops, some of the major high street shops now have computer sections and advice is readily available. For most people ease of use is essential. If records are to be kept on computer one needs to be able to call them onto the screen, correct or up-date, print out if necessary, and then store, with the minimum of fuss.

A suitable computer system for those in the horse business is available as a complete package, including the necessary programs, for under £1000 at current prices. The system consists of the central processing unit, the keyboard, a screen and a printer (hardware), together with word processing, management and financial programs (software). There are many accounting software packages available, some of them extremely complex. All that is needed is a program that will cover revenue, expenditure and balance sheet accounts, and VAT (including the cash accounting scheme). Most programs will cope with all normal routine transactions, including such essentials as bank reconciliations. Many calculations can be performed automatically – for example, balances against budget and totals for the current period against last year's totals for the same period. Other programs for the computer can handle stud records, riding school bookings and so on.

Reliability of the complete package and back-up service is important, and it is probably best to enter into a service agreement with the retailer. In fact, personal computers are generally very reliable, and become more sophisticated every day.

Most important of all is to make time to train all relevant staff in the use of the system.

Communications

The telephone is another vital piece of equipment, and a wide choice is available. A cordless telephone is extremely useful; it will operate around the yard and so can be answered even when riding! If, to answer an inquiry, it is necessary to consult someone else or look at the records, the conversation can be continued whilst looking for the person or file. Cordless telephones are inexpensive and easy to install.

It is also worth considering installing a robust, well-placed extension in the stables or riding school. A telephone answering machine is essential for a business receiving impulse inquiries. For example, the owner of a brood mare may decide to telephone the owners of possible stallions, and if the stallion owner is out will be able to leave a message. People are no longer so reluctant as they were to speak to a machine, and the initial cost is small. It is not worth hiring a telephone answering machine nowadays as such a small capital outlay is involved in purchasing one.

Mobile telephones are becoming commonplace; many horse professionals find they are invaluable for business; they also provide for speedy help to an incident if out trekking.

A fax is now inexpensive and allows notes, figures, diagrams and pictures to be sent down the telephone line.

Stationery

Good quality paper and envelopes and a well-designed letter heading provide a business with a good public image. Every communication conveys the image of the business. The first essential is to choose a 'house style' in colour of paper, type of print and possibly a logo. A logo is the emblem or symbol by which the business is recognized. It should be simple and easily recognizable, and all of its potential uses should be considered before a choice is made. The business logo should indicate not merely that it is an equestrian business, but also that it is *the* particular business. Well-known examples of logos in the horse world are the cocked hat of Wellington Riding and the stylized name of Warwickshire College.

The cost of professional design and layout is relatively small, and a design service is offered by most of the national printing franchises as well as by many ordinary printers.

The chosen colour for the notepaper or the colour and style of type should be used on all printed matter. It can also be carried through on the stable doors and paintwork. It should certainly be used on the business notice-board at the entrance to the premises where the name and business logo can be proudly displayed.

Insurance

Every business needs insurance and it may be convenient to find an insurance broker who will advise and arrange the cover which is needed. Insurance broking is now strictly controlled, but it is still up to the owner to decide on the extent of cover required and the 'best buys'. The National Farmers' Union offers a comprehensive service to its members and has local agents to give advice. A business affiliated to the British Horse Society or another organization may find that there are especially advantageous insurance services arranged through the organization's specialist brokers. Certain insurance is compulsory, e.g. under the Employers' Liability (Compulsory Insurance) Act 1969 which requires all employees to be covered for any injury they may suffer in the course of their employment and under the Riding Establishments Act 1964 for third party liability sustained while clients are riding or receiving instruction.

The many types of insurance may be put together in a comprehensive policy covering many eventualities – vehicles, employers' liability, public liability, personal insurance, horses and premises.

Vehicles

Third party insurance cover for every motor vehicle using the public roads is mandatory. It covers damage to other vehicles and people when there is liability. More valuable vehicles are usually insured comprehensively so as to cover the cost of repair or replacement in case of an accident. In addition it may be sensible to take out membership of one of the national breakdown help and 'get you home' schemes: this is a form of insurance. If a vehicle carries 'goods' for 'hire or reward', it must be licensed either for 'farmers'-goods' or as a haulier's vehicle. This is essential if, as is normal, livery clients are charged for transport to competitions or hunting. Infringement of the regulations or of the obligations involved in the licences is an offence and failure to comply with the terms of the licence may mean that the insurers are not liable.

Employers' liability

This is compulsory in respect of all employees in case they are injured or pick up certain diseases whilst carrying out their work. Working with horses is a high risk occupation. The amount of cover must be at least £2 million in respect of claims arising out of any one occurrence, but many policies give unlimited cover. The Employers' Liability Certificate must legally be displayed where the staff can see it, e.g. on the office wall. It is a criminal offence not to display the certificate.

Public liability

Any establishment open to the public should take out public liability insurance to cover potential liabilities to members of the public who may be injured. Riding establishments seeking a licence must establish that they are properly insured against liability for injuries sustained by riders and injured third parties. A stud having an open day or a school holding a gymkhana can take out suitable insurance to cover just that event.

Insurance policies of this type usually contain specific conditions which must be observed if the cover is not to be invalidated. (Any insurance policy received should be read with great care to find out exactly what is covered and also the particular terms and conditions.) A common requirement is that all riders must wear properly fitted hard hats to the current British Standard specification. In that case, a groom riding with the hat's chin strap unsecured might possibly be uninsured because modern hats must have a secured chin strap. Similarly, if a client is hired or loaned a hard hat, it must be of current BSI specification and correctly fitted and worn. An instructor should always check that this is the case and make the necessary adjustments.

Both the terms of insurance and the owner's legal liability under the law of negligence require that proprietors of equestrian businesses should warn the public of the potential risks involved with horses. It is no longer possible to exempt oneself from negligence liability resulting in death or personal injury, but in certain circumstances the law recognizes that voluntary assumption of the risks involved may amount to a defence to an action for damage or injury brought against the person responsible.

It is therefore a sensible precaution to have suitable warning notices on the premises. One should state simply: 'All visitors should report to reception on arrival'. A second notice, in the reception area, should be along the following lines:

(1) Horses kick, bite and move quickly in certain circumstances so take proper care.
(2) Do not go near to the horses unless supervised by staff.
(3) All clients must read and follow our safety code.

The safety code should also be displayed.

By this means, clients and visitors are warned in advance, and there is thus less chance of someone getting injured. If someone were injured, then adequate warnings of these sort could well mitigate potential liability.

Personal insurance

Those who work for themselves should be adequately insured. They may need to employ someone else to do the work if they are ill, and they may require protection against loss of income. Various assurances of this type are available and any competent broker will be able to advise. A personal accident policy will pay a set amount each week for a stated period; other policies pay until normal retirement age. Additionally, the self-employed may need private health insurance tailored to their special needs. Private health insurance is not expensive and there are various types of policy. Most of them cover hospital accommodation charges, surgeons' and other fees and expenses, and some provide a cash benefit as well.

The self-employed should also consider taking out a personal pension policy and tax relief is available on the premiums. Some policies are linked to equity investments or unit trusts, but all of them offer an option on retirement of a fixed sum each month or of a lump sum and a reduced pension. They can also have provision for a surviving spouse. As the rules are changing constantly, the advice of an accountant should be obtained before a decision is made.

Many businesses operate partly on money borrowed from a bank or other financial institution, whether the borrowings are secured by a mortgage or not. It is often a condition of such loans that the borrower should take out a personal life insurance and the costs are variable. Some policies are initially expensive but reduce in cost as the term proceeds; others have a fixed rate throughout their duration. The choice is a matter of personal needs and bank managers and accountants are useful advisers.

Horses

Insuring a horse shares the risk of losing it. Insurance is available to cover accidents and injuries to or sickness and disease of horses and ponies as well as their loss by theft or straying. In some cases, the loss of a horse may be covered by a more general policy, e.g. in a building contents policy which may, dependent on its terms, cover against the loss of livestock through fire. It is a matter of commercial judgment as to whether horses are worth insuring especially as the cost can be quite high. Horses of exceptional merit may well be worth insuring and individual owners may wish to insure their horses both for loss and for loss of use. This last-named type of insurance costs more than the conventional policy, but if it is taken out the insurers will pay a percentage of the horse's value if it becomes incapable of doing the specified activity. Policies may also cover such items as loss or theft of tack and veterinary expenses – usually as optional extras. An important consideration for all riders (whether in business or not) is to have cover against any accident involving a third party or parties. A runaway horse or one out of control can do a great deal of damage, and its owner could face a substantial claim if negligence is established.

Premises

As with domestic premises, business premises should be insured against the usual risks such as damage by fire, exceptional weather conditions and so on. Contents will need separate insurance. It is sensible to insure hay or straw in storage. Tack is expensive and is a high-risk item and should also be insured. Even if insured, loss of tack causes a great deal of inconvenience and so it is worth taking precautions to see that it is safe. Precautions may include a burglar alarm and other warning systems. Many insurance companies set specific requirements for the security of tackroom doors and windows. A useful source of free advice is the Crime Prevention Officer from the local police force.

Accounting procedures

Petty cash

Major items, such as a new saddle, should be paid for by cheque against an invoice, thus providing a record of the transaction which will be entered in the cash analysis book. Smaller items, however, can be paid for in cash, and cash transactions must be strictly controlled. A sensible petty cash system is to have a 'float' of (say) £100 in a locking cash box, the money being drawn by cheque from the bank and 'petty cash' being entered on the cheque counterfoil. As cash payments are made, they are marked in a petty cash book which is kept with the box. Business expenses paid for in cash out of one's own pocket when away from the yard are also reimbursed from the same fund, and the relevant entry is made in the book. Receipts should always be obtained if possible. When the cash float is running low, it is topped up by way of cash from the bank, and the petty cash book and contents of the box should be reconciled.

An alternative method of petty cash control is to use the imprest system, whereby at the end of each month the float is made up by exactly the right amount so as to restore the opening figure.

Book-keeping: the cash analysis account

All business enterprises must keep an accurate record of all receipts and payments during the financial year. An accountant can advise on the appropriate system, but if the accounts are kept manually (and not on computer) a simple procedure is best. A well-tried system is based on the use of the single entry or cash analysis account book in which all receipts and payments of money are entered as received or made. The book is divided into columns so that items can be classified; receipts are entered on one page, and payments on another. The figures are totalled monthly and then can be reconciled with the bank statements. The headings of each column will depend on the nature of the enterprise, but a typical equine business might use:

Receipts
Livery fees
Instruction
Sale of horses
Transport charges
Sundries

Payments
Hay and straw
Concentrates
Transport costs
Insurances
Wages and National Insurance
Rates
Mortgage repayments
Bank charges and interest
Subscriptions

In both cases there should be columns for value added tax (VAT).

One book is kept for each business year, and the loose-leaf form may be found most convenient. The book (or the pages for the year) are submitted to the accountant at the end of the year together with all supporting records – the petty cash book, wages book, receipts, invoices and the like – so that the business accounts can be audited for submission to the Inland Revenue. The accountant will prepare the business's profit and loss account, which will include other items such as depreciation of equipment and, of course, the audit fee.

Using this system means that only two other books are essential: the petty cash book and a wages book. The wages book shows the details of each employee's weekly earnings, with columns for gross wages, nett wages, income tax deducted and the employee's share of National Insurance contributions. The weekly total of the gross wages is then transferred to the cash analysis book; income tax and National Insurance contributions (including the employer's share) will be sent by cheque to the Collector of Taxes in due course, and the employer's share of the National Insurance is also entered in the cash analysis book as a labour cost. This method involves the minimum of effort and the only other essential book-keeping records are the bank statements, cheque book counterfoils (properly filled in!) and stubs of the in-payment slips. Since the majority of banks no longer give itemized statements showing the person to whom payments have been made, it is wise to record the number of any cheque against the appropriate entry. If any payments are made by bank standing order these should not be forgotten.

All payments and receipts should go through the bank account, and thus the cash analysis book and bank statements will match up, provided that any bank charges are entered into the cash analysis book. The bank is the one trader who fails to send a bill! The money kept in the current account should be the minimum needed for trading (and to avoid bank charges). Any surplus funds should be placed on a deposit account so as to earn interest, although the banks are now moving to the situation where interest will be paid on current accounts too.

The bank is often a good source of business advice and many branches have specialist business advisors.

Monthly totalling of the cash analysis book is essential. The monthly totals should be made when the bank statements are received, and the totals will be adjusted to allow for any uncleared cheques. Thus, the owner is able to keep an eye on the financial health of the business. Most equine businesses will be registered for VAT and this involves the regular submission of VAT returns to the Commissioners of Customs and Excise, usually accompanied by a payment of the difference between the VAT input tax (which has been charged to the business by suppliers) and the output tax (which has been charged by the business to its clients).

When ordering goods, after receiving and considering any quotations, an order is written and then the delivery note and invoice can be reconciled with the order. Payment is made by cheque and the amount is shown as an expense in the appropriate column of the cash analysis book. If goods are sold – a horse, for example – an invoice should be raised showing the amount of VAT. This is then entered as a receipt in the book. Any cash transactions, e.g. riding lessons, must also be recorded. A riding school dealing largely with cash clients should keep a till and check the takings at the end of each day. These are then paid into the bank on a regular basis, and the paying-in slip provides the record for the entry made in the cash analysis book. Payments should never be made from the till but always from petty cash.

Two other areas are slightly more complex – veterinary expenses and farrier's charges. The best plan is to have a duplicate book for each of these kept in the yard, listing the horses and any treatment or shoeing. Each book is completed at the time of the visit, and the duplicate sheet is taken to the office to be reconciled with the account. The stable manager of a livery yard should keep similar books for recording things such as clipping and worming which are chargeable to the client. This procedure sounds complicated but is simple to operate in practice. The most common mistake is that services are simply not recorded.

The end of the financial year

At the end of each financial year there are other accounting procedures to be carried out, usually by the accountant from the books and records kept by the business throughout the year: valuation, the profit and loss account, and the balance sheet.

Valuation

The whole business should be valued at the close of the year, usually on the last financial day of the year. Valuation means a formal assessment of the worth of the assets of the business, and starts off with an inventory. Valuation is a profession and so only general guidance can be given; the small business owner will rely on the accountant for advice because the tax implications of the net capital of the business must be borne in mind. The valuation should be realistic. Stock can be valued at the cost of production or at its estimated market value – the price it would fetch if sold in the open market under normal conditions. For tax purposes, if the actual costs of production cannot be accurately shown, the Inland Revenue authorities will usually allow stock which is to be sold on (trading livestock) to be valued at current market value, less an agreed percentage. If the value of stock is over-estimated (i.e. valued above what it cost to produce), the business will appear to be making a profit on paper, although the 'profit' will not in fact exist. It is foolish to value on the basis of anticipated profits. To avoid a 'paper profit' it is best to be conservative in valuing both young stock and competition animals. In valuing machines and implements, one starts with the previous year's total value, adds in the value of items purchased and deducts any items sold. An allowance is made for depreciation at the rate agreed with the accountant – and this is usually 25 per cent. Stores in stock are shown at cost price, regardless of current market value, e.g. hay in the barn is shown in the accounts at the price it was bought in at, regardless of any increase in value. Small items – such as bits – are usually 'written off' in the year of purchase.

Trading and profit and loss account

This shows the amount of profit (or loss) made over the year, and so is an important tool for financial management. It is mainly based on the information provided by the cash analysis account. The expenses of the business (adjusted for any difference between the opening and closing value of stocks held by the business) are deducted from the sales for the year, to leave the figure of net profit. If the expenses are greater than the sales, then the business has made a net loss. The calculation is usually made in two stages:

Sales	minus	*cost of sales* (the direct costs of feed, bedding, vet, stock purchases, etc., adjusted for changes in stock values)	= *Gross profit*
Gross profit	minus	*overhead expenses* (labour, rent and rates, vehicle expenses, administration and finance costs)	= *Net profit*

The balance sheet

A complete financial picture at the end of each year is provided by the balance sheet:

Liabilities		Assets	
		Valuation of business	
Debts payable – goods and services received but not yet paid for, i.e. money owed to creditors	£	Debts due – goods and services sold but not yet paid for, i.e. money owed by debtors	£
Bank overdraft	£	Money in the bank	£
Borrowed money, e.g. mortgage debts	£	Cash in hand	£
Total liabilities:	£‾‾‾	Total assets:	£‾‾‾
Net capital: £			

Both sides must balance. The point of the exercise is to establish the value of the business on the day, i.e. its net capital. If this comes to a negative figure, the business is insolvent.

5 The law

Introduction

A basic knowledge of business law is an essential part of management. 'Ignorance of the law is no excuse' and every aspect of business is affected by legal considerations. This chapter outlines some essential law.

English law consists of statute law – Acts of Parliament and regulations made under them such as the Importation of Equine Animals Order 1970 – and common law or case law. Common law is the rules and principles expressed in decisions of the courts over the centuries. Under the English system of case law, a judge is bound to decide a question in the way in which it has been decided previously by judges in one of the superior courts (the House of Lords, Court of Appeal or the High Court) in earlier cases. This is called the system of judicial precedent. Case law is a most important part of English law and grows on a daily basis.

For our purposes, there are two broad categories of law: civil (or private) law and criminal law. Civil law deals with the relationships between citizens; civil law duties can be enforced by litigation in a private action in the High Court or the County Court and are remedied by an order for the the payment of money compensation (damages) or some other remedy such as an injunction. In contrast, criminal law deals with offences against the public good and is enforced by prosecution by the State or its agents. If crime is established it can be punished by fine or imprisonment.

Civil law includes the law of contract and the law of tort, both of which are of great importance to owners of horse establishments. Contract deals with legally binding agreements between people, for example a contract of employment, a contract to buy a horse or a contract for the sale of land. The law of tort deals with civil wrongs where there is a breach of some duty imposed generally by the law. There are many types of torts such as negligence, trespass and private nuisance.

This chapter deals only in wide-ranging outline with some of the law affecting horse businesses. A useful book for reference is *Essential Law for Landowners and Farmers* by M. Gregory and A. Sydenham (Third edition, Blackwell Science), but wherever there is a legal problem the advice of a competent solicitor should be obtained.

The law of contract

All businesses involve buying and selling; contracts for the sale of goods are the most frequent business transaction. Contrary to popular opinion, a contract does not normally need to be in writing or be supported by written evidence except in special cases. These cases apart, a verbal contract is valid and enforceable, and any dispute is decided on the basis of the evidence before the court. Documentary evidence is often desirable, but the majority of day-to-day contracts are made by word of mouth, e.g. having a riding lesson in return for a fee or buying a beer in a public house. Generally, then, a contract does not need to be in any particular form, but there are important exceptions such as contracts of hire-purchase. These must be made in writing in a prescribed form under the Consumer Credit Act 1974.

Detailed consideration of the general law of contract is outside the scope of this book, but since buying and selling is such an important part of any business activity, something must be said about the rules governing sales of goods. Contracts for the sale of goods do not need to be in writing. 'Goods' include horses and other livestock as well as inanimate objects such as hay, machinery, vehicles, etc. They are governed by the Sale of Goods Act 1979. Section 2(1) of the Act defines a contract for the sale of goods as one 'by which the seller transfers or agrees to transfer the property in goods to the buyer for a money consideration, called the price'. A sale of goods therefore involves three essential elements: (a) a contract (b) a transfer of goods and (c) the price.

A contract

A contract is a legally binding agreement made between two or more parties. It involves an offer made by one party, unconditionally accepted by the other party, and supported by consideration, i.e. the price. The agreement must not be uncertain in any way and the application of this rule gives rise to many difficulties in practice. In one case, for example, a theatre manager agreed to engage an actress 'at a West End salary to be agreed between us'. It was ruled that there was no binding contract unless and until the parties agreed the salary.

A transfer of goods

Section 61(1) of the Sale of Goods Act 1979 contains a very complex definition of the simple word 'goods'. It includes not only animals but also growing crops or anything else which is attached to land, but which it is agreed will be detached. A typical equestrian example is the purchase of hay from the field.

The price

This is the payment in exchange for the goods. Transfer of ownership in the goods does not depend on the actual payment of the price. Ownership passes from the seller to the buyer when the parties intend it to be transferred and they are free to make appropriate provision in the contract. If, as is usually the case in the horse world, the parties make no express provision, s. 18 of the 1979 Act lays down specific rules. Two of them are of particular importance. The basic rule is that where there is a contract for the sale of specific goods in a deliverable state, such as a horse, 'the property in the goods passes to the buyer when the contract is made, and it is immaterial whether the time of payment or the time of delivery, or both, is postponed'. In the normal case, therefore, the ownership is transferred when the bargain is struck.

A different rule applies where goods are delivered to the buyer on approval or on sale or return or other similar terms. In that case, ownership is transferred when the buyer signifies approval or acceptance to the seller or does something else which makes it clear that he/she is adopting the transaction. The buyer cannot hold out indefinitely. If no time limit has been specified, then the buyer must act within what lawyers call 'a reasonable time'.

The law *implies* certain terms to be performed by the seller into contracts for the sale of goods. A most important term, which cannot be excluded, is that the seller has the right to sell and that in the case of an agreement to sell, the seller has the right to do so at the time ownership passes to the buyer: 1979 Act, s. 12(1)(a). For example, if a client agrees to buy a horse from a dealer and nothing is said about ownership, the buyer can assume that the dealer owns the horse or has the right to sell as agent or will have that right when ownership is transferred.

This is a condition of the contract – a term of vital importance – and if the dealer did not have the right to sell, the buyer could repudiate the contract and recover the purchase price. In some cases the buyer might also recover damages. In one case, a horse was sold by mistake at an auction. The mistake was discovered and delivery of the horse was refused to the buyer. The auctioneer who had mistakenly sold the horse was held liable to pay damages to the buyer.

Another implied condition applies where there is a sale by description, e.g. a saddle described as 'a jumping saddle'. The goods must then comply with the description, i.e. the saddle must be cut for jumping. If the goods do not do so, the buyer can sue for damages: 1979 Act, s. 13. The same rule applies where a horse is sold by description.

The common law rule of *caveat emptor* ('let the buyer beware') is restated by s. 14(1) of the 1979 Act. What it means is that the purchaser must be careful when buying goods and examine them for obvious defects. This basic rule applies to private sales but is modified for sales made *in the course of a business* when other terms are imposed. These cannot be excluded by the seller in 'consumer sales', i.e. sales made by a seller who is selling goods as a business to someone for private use and who is not buying in the course of a business. The classic example is a sale of a horse by a dealer or a riding stables to a private client.

The conditions implied are: (a) merchantable quality (b) fitness for purpose and (c) sale by sample.

Merchantable quality

Goods sold must be of 'merchantable quality'. This is defined as being as 'fit for the purpose(s) for which goods of that kind are commonly bought as it is reasonable to expect having regard to any description applied to them, the price (if relevant) and all the other relevant circumstances': 1979 Act, s. 14(2). The requirement applies to both new and second-hand goods, although if goods are sold as second-hand, the buyer must expect goods of a lower standard.

The application of this rule to a sale of new goods is shown by a case in 1987 where a new Range Rover had a defective engine, gearbox, bodywork and oil seals. Each of these defects required repairs, but none of them made the vehicle unroadworthy or undrivable. It was nonetheless held that the vehicle was not of merchantable quality. The court rejected the argument that one should expect some defects in a new vehicle and that the Range Rover was not unmerchantable because there was a manufacturer's warranty. This was irrelevant to the contractual position between the buyer and the seller.

In another case, the contract was for the sale of a second-hand car. The engine failed after 2,300 miles of use by the buyer. The car was held not to have been of merchantable quality.

There are two exceptions to the rule about merchantable quality:

- It does not apply if the defects are drawn specifically to the buyer's attention before the contract is made.
- It does not apply where the buyer actually examines the goods before the contract is made as regards defects which the buyer's examination ought to reveal.

Fitness for purpose

If the buyer makes known to the seller the purpose for which the goods are required, either by telling the seller expressly or by implication, there is an implied condition that the goods will be fit for that purpose, unless the circumstances show that the buyer is not relying on the seller's skill or judgement or that it would be unreasonable for the buyer to do so: 1979 Act, s. 14(3).

In the horse world, buyers often rely on the seller's skill and judgement when purchasing a horse. The purpose does not have to be explained to the buyer if it is obvious what the horse is going to be used for. Two examples illustrate the situation. A rider approaches a dealer and says that he requires a horse for jumping and is sold a horse that does not jump. There is a breach of the condition. A novice rider approaches the riding school where he is receiving lessons and says that he wants to buy a horse. He is sold a very fiery mount which is hard to control. There would again be a breach of the condition.

Sale by sample

Under s. 15 of the 1979 Act, where goods are ordered by reference to a sample, there is an implied condition that the bulk will correspond with the sample. The buyer must be given a reasonable opportunity to check this.

This rule is important when buying hay, straw and so on where there is often a sale by sample. If the bulk supplied is not of the right quality then the buyer can reject the goods and recover the purchase price.

The condition about title (s. 12) can never be excluded from a contract of sale. The last three conditions mentioned cannot be excluded by the seller in 'consumer sales' which is of importance to equestrian businesses which sell horses, etc. to clients as part of the business. It applies even if the business has only just started.

Express warranties and conditions

Apart from the terms implied by the Sale of Goods Act 1979, many sales of horses are subject to express warranties and undertakings given by the seller to the buyer. Statements that a horse is 'warranted sound', 'warranted sound in wind and limb', 'warranted as a good hunter', 'warranted free from vice' or 'warranted quiet in every way' are all express warranties. They are conditions of the contract. If the statements prove untrue, the condition is broken. The purchaser is then entitled to repudiate the contract within a reasonable time and get his/her money back on returning the horse and to claim damages. Express warranties only cover the position at the time of sale, but as will be seen there is a broad legal definition of 'unsoundness'. Case law establishes that the seller is liable if he/she warrants a horse as 'sound' and it later proves to be unsound because of some latent defect.

A warranty may be limited in time as is usually the case at auction sales of horses where there are special conditions covering warranties given in the catalogue descriptions or by the auctioneer. The usual condition is that notice of the alleged breach must be given within a short time period and that any dispute is to be decided by an independent veterinary surgeon. Once the period specified has elapsed, the right to complain of the breach of condition is lost. It is best to follow a similar practice if selling a horse in the course of one's own business.

There is a distinction between unsoundness and vice. Unsoundness is a question of usefulness and not of disease. In the words of a nineteenth century judge:

> 'The rule as to unsoundness is that if at the time of sale, the horse has any disease which either actually does diminish the natural usefulness of the animal, so as to make him less capable of work of any description or which in its ordinary progress will diminish the natural usefulness of the animal, or if the horse has, either from disease or accident undergone any alterations of structure that either actually does at the time, or in its ordinary effects will, diminish the natural usefulness of the horse, such a horse is unsound': Baron Parke in *Coates* v. *Stephens* (1838).

This old definition is important. In practice, it may be apparent that at the time of sale a horse has a disease or defect which diminishes its natural usefulness, but it is very difficult to establish whether a horse has some minor defect which may diminish its natural usefulness in the future which again makes the animal unsound. This is one of the reasons why veterinary surgeons do not like to certify a horse as 'sound'.

Broken wind, coughing, navicular disease, spavin and wind galls producing lameness have all been held to be instances of unsoundness, and there are many others.

A vice – contrasted with unsoundness – is a particular habit or temperament in the animal which is not ordinarily found in a horse, and which has the effect of rendering it dangerous or less useful or liable to suffer in health. Kicking and crib-biting are typical instances of vice.

Misrepresentation

In negotiations leading up to a sale, the seller often makes statements about his/her wares which do not become terms of the contract. Sometimes the statements are mere 'puffs' not intended to be taken seriously; in other cases there are statements of fact which are one of the significant inducing causes of the contract but which fall short of becoming terms of the contract. Untrue statements of this sort are called misrepresentations, and the party who has been misled may be able to claim damages and/or treat the contract as at an end if he/she can establish that he/she was induced to enter into the contract because of the misrepresentation. The misstatement must be one of fact, not of pure opinion or of law. But a seller cannot escape liability merely by prefacing a statement with 'I believe that', or 'In my opinion', especially where the seller is in the trade.

Misrepresentations are either fraudulent, innocent or negligent. A fraudulent misrepresentation is a false statement of fact made 'knowingly, or without belief in its truth, or recklessly, careless whether it to be true or false', i.e. dishonestly: *Derry* v. *Peek* (1889). Proving that a statement is fraudulent is difficult. A negligent misrepresentation is easier to establish. It is a careless statement of fact made in circumstances which make it likely that the other person will reasonably rely on it. This will invariably be the case where the seller of goods is a trader. An innocent misrepresentation is an untrue statement made without fault on the part of the maker.

A fraudulent misrepresentation entitles the innocent party to claim damages and to have the contract set aside. Alternatively, he/she may claim damages for deceit and affirm the contract. Someone who has been induced to enter into a contract by a negligent misrepresentation can set the contract aside on discovering the truth and/or claim damages. The maker of a negligent misrepresentation must pay damages unless able to prove that he/she has reasonable grounds to believe and did believe up to the time the contract was made that the facts represented were true. If the contract is induced by an innocent misrepresentation, the person misled may also rescind the contract or obtain damages in lieu at the discretion of the court. There are some limits to the right to set the contract aside, but this is a broad summary of the position.

Contracts of employment

Contracts of employment can be entered into formally or informally. (An example of a formal contract is that for a working pupil, as discussed below.) They usually come about as a result of interviews as discussed in Chapter 3 when the parties should expressly agree the terms which form the basis of the contract: nature of the duties, hours of work, holidays, overtime, time off, sick pay and so on. If the employer provides facilities for an employee's property, e.g. car parking or a cloakroom, the employer cannot restrict his/her liability for death or injury resulting from negligence, and as a result of s. 2 of the Unfair Contract Terms Act 1977 the employer can only exclude or restrict his/her liability for damage to the employee's property by a term of the contract which is reasonable in all the circumstances.

Every employee who works for at least eight hours a week must be given a written statement of the terms and conditions of his/her employment within two months of starting work. It is not sufficient for employees to be told or shown the terms of employment: they must be given a document for reference purposes. The Trade Union and Employment Rights Act 1993 says that this statement may be given in instalments before the end of the two month period, but in small establishments it is sensible to give a complete written statement no later than one month after the person starts work.

The statutory written statement must contain the following information:

- The names of the parties.
- The date when the employment began and the date on which the employee's period of continuous employment began (taking into account any previous employment with a previous employer).
- The rate or scale of remuneration or method of calculating it.
- The intervals at which it is to be paid, e.g. weekly or monthly.
- The terms and conditions relating to hours of work, including normal working hours.

- Terms and conditions of holiday entitlement (including public holidays), holiday pay and accrued holiday pay.
- Details of any sick pay or pension rights.
- The length of notice which the employee must give and is entitled to receive.
- The title of the job the employee is employed to do or a brief job description.
- Where the employment is not intended to be permanent, the period for which it is expected to continue. If the job is for a fixed term, the statement must say so.
- The place of work. If the employee will work at several places, this must be indicated and the employer's address must be stated.

Collective (Union) agreements directly affecting terms and conditions of employment must also be specified and extra detail is required where the employee is required to work outside the UK for a month or more. These two requirements will affect few, if any, equine establishments.

Obviously, any changes must also be notified as well, and the provisions do not apply to anyone whose employment continues for less than one month. Most people do not find the legal requirements too onerous in practice, even though they grumble about the paperwork!

If you employ twenty people or more, then every employee who works at least eight hours a week is entitled to an itemized pay statement as well. Although this is a legal requirement, it is sensible management practice in any business, however small.

The statutory written statement is not the contract between the parties but is strong evidence of what the contract terms are. This statement should be prepared in duplicate and the employee should be asked to sign one copy which should be kept in his/her employment file. The statement must also include a note:

- specifying any disciplinary rules applicable to the employee or referring to a document such as a Staff Handbook which specifies those rules and which is reasonably accessible to the employee;
- specifying by name or description the person to whom the employee can apply if he/she feels dissatisfied with any disciplinary decision;
- specifying the person to whom the employee can apply if he/she has a grievance about his/her employment.

This is not as formidable as it sounds and printed pro-forma written particulars can be obtained from most stationers. What is more problematical is the fact that, whatever has been agreed about notice from the employer bringing the contract of employment to an end, all employees who have been continuously employed for more than one year are protected from *unfair dismissal*, which can occur even if the employer terminates the contract with notice or pay in lieu of notice. Every employee covered by the legislation has the right not to be unfairly dismissed, and the remedy is for the employee to complain to an industrial tribunal, which has power to award compensation. Although there is no dismissal if the employee agrees to resign, there will be a dismissal if an employee is threatened with dismissal unless he does resign.

There are five main grounds on which a dismissal is capable of being fair:

- The reason relates to the capability or qualifications of the employee for performing the work of the kind which he/she was employed to do.
- It relates to the conduct of the employee.
- Redundancy. In this case the employee may be entitled to redundancy pay, the amount of which is dependent on age, length of service and the amount of the weekly pay.
- Because the employee cannot continue to work in the position held without contravening some statutory obligation, e.g. where an employee who is required to drive motor vehicles loses his/her driving licence.
- There is some other substantial reason justifying the dismissal.

Provided the dismissal is on one of these grounds and that the proper procedures have been observed so that there is a full investigation, a proper hearing, a right to appeal and so on (as set out in the ACAS Code of Practice, which is obtainable from Her Majesty's Stationery Office) the dismissal will be held to be fair. In reaching a decision to dismiss, the employer must consider all the circumstances. The dismissal will be fair if the employer has acted reasonably, but the employer is not the best person to decide whether he or she has been 'reasonable'. When in doubt consult a solicitor.

Working pupil contracts

The position of working pupils requires brief consideration because many riding schools and stables operate a working pupil scheme under which the establishment offers practical and theoretical tuition for examinations in return for fees and the working pupil carrying out specific duties. The trade unions' opposition to the system has some justification in practice because, in the past, the system has been abused and working pupils have been used as a form of cheap labour.

The British Horse Society has made various recommendations about the points which should be covered in a working pupil contract and agreed by the establishment and the pupil before the course commences. These recommendations are not mandatory and are merely a guide and, of course, do not have the effect of law. They are merely recommendations. The BHS suggests that the contract should include:

- a broad description of the duties which the working pupil is expected to perform;
- financial arrangements;
- details of any probationary period;
- hours of work;
- public and other holidays and time off, which should include weekends;
- the mounted and dismounted training which the working pupil will receive, including practical teaching experience;
- the examination for which the training will be given, its approximate date, and responsibility for making the entry;
- food and accommodation, including bedding, linen, etc.;
- keep of working pupil's horse (if any);
- competitions, hunting, etc;
- disciplinary rules, e.g. time-keeping, dress, etc. A working pupil contract should be entered into formally between the establishment and the student and his/her parents. A specimen contract is available from the BHS.

The law of tort

A tort is a civil wrong other than a breach of contract or a breach of trust which gives rise to an action for damages or some other civil remedy. It is not a criminal wrong and is not punishable by the State. Each tort has developed separately and has its own characteristics and remedies. Important torts include negligence, trespass and private nuisance, all of which are of importance to the occupier of land.

Negligence

Negligence in law is not the same as carelessness or mistake: it is conduct and not a state of mind. Negligence is the breach of a duty of care owed by one person to another which results in damage. It is the omission to do something that a reasonable man would do, or the doing of something that a prudent and reasonable man would not do. To succeed in an action for negligence, the plaintiff (claimant) must establish:

(a) that the defendant was under a duty of care owed to the plaintiff. Everyone has a duty to take reasonable care not to harm others;
(b) that the defendant was in breach of that duty;
(c) that the plaintiff suffered foreseeable damage as a result. 'Damage' usually means physical harm to persons or property but in rare cases it can include purely financial loss.

There is a large and, unfortunately, fast growing body of case law dealing with negligence and there is no way in which an equestrian establishment can exclude or limit liability for *death or personal injury resulting from negligence* because of the provisions of the Unfair Contract Terms Act 1977 which is as crucial to tort as it is to contract. The Act applies to 'business liability', i.e. liability arising from 'things done or to be done by a person in the course of a business' and the occupation of premises used for 'business purposes'. Any contract term or notice purporting to exclude liability will be invalid. In the case of other loss caused by negligence, or death or personal injury resulting from a tort other than negligence, an exclusion or limitation of liability is a nullity unless it satisfies a vague test of 'reasonableness'. Clearly, then, the display by a riding establishment of a notice saying 'Clients ride entirely at their own risk' is ineffective to protect the proprietor. Warning notices are still desirable, however, as indications that the owner of the business has acted prudently.

It is important to realize that an employer is vicariously liable for the actions of employees acting in the course of employment even if the employee is acting in defiance of an express prohibition. Adequate insurance cover against civil liability is therefore essential.

Voluntary assumption of risk

The Latin maxim *volenti non fit injuria* (where there is consent there is no injury) provides a very limited defence to an action in tort in very special circumstances. Those who take part in a sport or pastime are sometimes taken to have accepted the risk of dangers which are incidental to the ordinary conduct of the pastime. It must be established that the claimant freely and voluntarily assumed the risk, with the full knowledge of its nature and extent. The maxim has little or no application to actions by employees against employers because a person employed as a servant who accepts a risk incidental to his/her employment is not to be treated as accepting it voluntarily. The 1977 Act previously discussed, further restricts its operation. In one case in 1962 it was applied where a non-paying spectator was injured by a horse competing at a jumping show. The rider was not liable even though he committed an error of judgement.

The Occupiers' Liability Acts 1957 and 1984

Negligence is generally applicable to activities being carried out on a property. These statutes set out the legal duty owed by the occupier of premises to 'visitors' (as defined) and to 'persons other than his visitors'. They are concerned with premises which are dangerous because they are in a defective or dangerous state. In some cases an injured person can sue alternatively for negligence and breach of the Act. The word 'premises' is defined in very wide terms and means the property of the occupier, including fixed or movable structures.

The 1957 Act applies to lawful visitors 'using the premises' and covers people entering with permission or at the invitation of the occupier, as well as people entering as of right such as the host of officials empowered by statute to enter premises. Permission may be express or implied, and so the definition covers all people lawfully on the property. Other entrants *including trespassers* are covered by the 1984 Act.

The 1957 Act provides that the occupier owes a 'common duty of care' to all visitors except to the limited extent that he/she can modify it by agreement. Section 2(2) defines the duty owed in these terms:

> 'The common duty of care as a duty to take such care as in all the circumstances of the case is reasonable to see that the visitor will be reasonably safe in using the premises for the purposes for which he is invited or permitted by the occupier to be there.'

Whether the standard required has been attained is a question of fact; the Act requires occupiers to act reasonably. The occupier must be prepared for children to be less careful than adults and what is not a danger to an adult may be a danger to a child. Adult visitors are expected to take reasonable care of themselves and where someone comes on to the property to exercise a calling, e.g. a window cleaner, they may be expected to appreciate and guard against any special risks ordinarily incidental to their job. If there are dangers on the premises the occupier should guard them. Visitors' attention should be drawn to any special or hidden dangers by suitable notices or other means. A warning does not of itself absolve from liability but will be taken into account in deciding whether the occupier is liable for a mishap.

Liability to trespassers and other uninvited entrants is regulated by s. 1 of the 1984 Act. A duty is owed to an uninvited entrant 'to take such care as is reasonable in all the circumstances of the case to see that he does not suffer injury (i.e. death or physical or mental injury, not property damage) on the premises by reason of the danger concerned' if three conditions are met:

(1) The occupier knows of the danger or has reasonable grounds to believe it exists.
(2) The occupier knows, or has reasonable grounds to believe, that the entrant either is or might come into the vicinity of the danger.
(3) The risk of injury resulting from the danger is one against which in all the circumstances of the case the occupier can reasonably be expected to offer the uninvited entrant some protection.

A significant difference between the common duty of care owed under the 1957 Act to visitors and the duty under the 1984 Act is that the latter can 'in an appropriate case, be discharged by taking such steps as are reasonable in all the circumstances of the case to give warning of the danger concerned or to discourage a person from incurring risk'. All this is very vague and while a plain warning notice might well discharge liability to adult trespassers, it would probably be ineffective in the case of mischievous children.

The Animals Act 1971

People who own and control animals are under the same duty of care as those responsible for anything else. In one case, for example, the defendant was held liable when his unattended pony became restive and grabbed at a passing pedestrian and dragged her down. Most of the law about liability for animals is now found in the Animals Act 1971, which imposes strict liability (i.e. liability without fault) on the keeper of an animal of a 'dangerous species' for any damage done by it. A dangerous species is one which is not commonly domesticated in the British Isles, and which, when fully grown, has such characteristics that it is likely, unless restrained, to cause severe damage or that any damage it may cause is likely to be severe.

Of more interest to the horse business is the liability imposed in certain circumstances on an animal which does not belong to a dangerous species: 1971 Act, s. 2(2). Horses and ponies fall into this grouping. Liability is imposed regardless of fault provided three requirements are met:

- The damage must be of a kind which the animal was likely to cause if not restrained, or which if caused by the animal was likely to be severe.
- The likelihood of the damage or its being severe must be due to characteristics of the animal which are not normally found in animals of the same species except at particular times or in particular circumstances.
- Those characteristics must be known to the keeper of the animal or his/her employee or to a member of his/her household over 16.

The situation is illustrated by a case in 1962, where a groom recovered damages from her employer where a horse of unpredictable and unreliable behaviour crushed her against the bar of its trailer. The horse, a thoroughbred show jumper, had no previous tendency to injure people, but the judge found that its characteristics were of a kind not normally found in horses and that its keeper knew all about its characteristics.

Section 4 of the Animals Act 1971 also imposes strict liability for damage done by straying livestock which trespass on to someone else's land. Livestock means cattle, horses, asses, mules, hinnies, sheep, pigs, goats and poultry, as well as deer not in the wild state. The liability is for damage done by the livestock to the land or any property on it, but not personal injuries. Liability is strict; no fault has to be proved, but if the damage is the fault of the person suffering it there is no liability. However, it is the animals' owner's obligation to keep his/her livestock in and not the responsibility of other owners to keep them out. It is also a defence if the livestock strayed from the highway and the livestock's presence there was a lawful use of the highway.

The person trespassed against has the right to detain and eventually sell livestock which stray on his/her land, and the animal's owner is liable to pay any expenses incurred in his/her doing so.

Section 8(1) of the 1971 Act imposes a duty of care to prevent animals straying on to the highway, but liability is not strict. The owner is not liable unless he/she has failed to exercise reasonable care to prevent the livestock straying, e.g. by fencing. But it is not a breach of the duty of care to place animals on unfenced common land where fencing is not customary, e.g. in the exercise of grazing rights on Dartmoor. If animals lawfully on the highway stray from it and cause damage, negligence must also be proved.

Trespass to land

Direct entry onto someone else's land without consent or lawful authority is trespass. Mistake, as such, is no defence to trespass. The occupier may sue even if no damage is done but this is seldom worthwhile. If a trespasser declines to leave the land when asked to do so, the law allows the occupier to eject the trespasser using no more force than is reasonably necessary, but it is very unwise to resort to self-help.

The Criminal Justice Bill allows the police to evict potential saboteurs from private land. Aggrevated trespass occurs when a person invades land to disrupt lawful activity.

Private nuisance

A private nuisance is a state of affairs which has been defined by the courts as 'an unlawful interference with a person's use or enjoyment of land or some right over or in connection with it'. The interference must be substantial and in general actual damage must be proved. Excessive noise, fumes, smells and so on have all been held to amount to nuisances; a muck heap might be held to amount to a nuisance as might the noise and smell from horses or other animals. Much depends on the character of the locality: in country districts some noise and smell from animals must be tolerated. But it is a question of degree and in one case a pig farmer used a field near a housing estate for the deposit of pig excrement. Much of the field was covered with slurry to a depth of 1 to 1.5 inches and the tipping had been carried out within close proximity of the windows of the houses causing personal discomfort to residents. This was held to amount to a nuisance. In essence whether or not something amounts to a nuisance is a matter of reasonableness and common sense. The characteristic remedy for private nuisance is an action for damages although the court may also grant an injunction which is an order to stop the nuisance.

Nuisance and trespass do not overlap, but there is an overlap between private nuisance and the rule in *Rylands* v. *Fletcher* (1886) which imposes strict liability on an occupier who brings something onto his/her land or accumulates it there and it escapes and causes damage. The bulk storage of water and the like has been held to be a 'non-natural use of land' for the purposes of the rule. There are very few defences to an action brought for damage caused by the escape.

(*Note*: Local authorities have powers to deal with 'statutory nuisances' by serving abatement notices enforced by orders made by the magistrates' court.)

The Riding Establishments Acts 1964 and 1970

Any equestrian establishment which hires out horses or gives riding lessons by way of business falls under this legislation, even if the activity is carried out only part-time. A licence must be obtained from the district council and the applicant must meet a number of conditions:

- The applicant must be a body corporate or at least 18 years of age.
- The applicant must not be disqualified from keeping a riding stable, a dog, pet shop, boarding kennels or from having custody of animals.
- The applicant must satisfy the local authority of his/her suitability and qualifications by examinations or experience to run a riding establishment. If the applicant holds an 'approved certificate' (such as even an Assistant Instructor's Certificate of the BHS), the need to prove experience of horse management is dispensed with.

Licences are granted on a provisional (three months) and annual basis, and before issuing the licence there is an inspection of the premises. The district council must take various matters into account in deciding whether or not to grant the licence, all of which are for the welfare and benefit of the horses: see Table 5.1.

The council may impose conditions to ensure that these requirements are met. Other basic conditions are:

- A horse found by an inspector to be in need of veterinary attention must not be returned to work until the licence owner has obtained and lodged with the council a veterinary certificate that the horse is fit for work.
- A horse must not be let out on hire for riding or used for providing riding instruction unless supervised by a responsible person aged over 15 unless the licence holder is satisfied that the hirer is competent to ride without supervision.
- There must always be a responsible person of at least 16 years of age in charge of the establishment during business hours.
- The licence holder must hold a current insurance policy covering him/her for personal injuries sustained by hirers or paying pupils and against injury to third parties arising from the hire or use of the horses.
- There must be a register of all horses in the licence holder's possession

Table 5.1 Matters which must be considered in deciding whether to grant a licence for a riding establishment.

Regard must be had to the need for securing that:

- Paramount consideration will be given to the condition of the horses and that they will be maintained in good health and in all respects physically fit.
- In the case of a horse kept for letting on hire or being used to provide riding instruction it will be suitable for its purpose.
- The feet of all animals are properly trimmed and that, if shod, the shoes are properly fitted and in good condition.
- There will be available at all times accommodation for horses which is suitable as respects size, construction, number of occupants, lighting, ventilation, drainage in both new and converted buildings.
- Where horses are kept at grass there will be available to them at all times adequate pasture, shelter and water and required supplementary feed.
- Horses will be adequately supplied with suitable food, drink and bedding material (if stabled).
- Horses will be adequately exercised, groomed and rested and visited at suitable intervals.
- All reasonable precautions will be taken to prevent and control the spread of infectious or contagious diseases among horses.
- Veterinary first aid equipment and medicines will be provided and maintained at the premises.
- Appropriate steps will be taken for the protection and extrication of horses in case of fire and in particular the name, address and telephone number of the licence holder or some other responsible person will be prominently displayed outside the premises.
- Instructions as to action to be taken in the event of fire will similarly be kept displayed.
- Adequate accommodation will be provided for forage, bedding, stable equipment and saddlery.

aged three years and under and usually kept on the premises. This register must be available for inspection by an authorized officer of the council at all times.

The annual inspections of most local authorities are very thorough, and the inspector (an authorized veterinary surgeon or veterinary practitioner) is empowered to inspect any premises in the district council's area where there is a licensed establishment or an establishment which has applied for a licence or where there is reason to believe that a person is keeping a riding establishment. This power is exercisable at all 'reasonable times'. Operating an unlicensed riding establishment is a criminal offence.

There are various other offences under the Acts. On conviction, the magistrates may fine or imprison the offender, and also disqualify the offender from holding a riding establishment licence.

The provisions of the Riding Establishments Acts are unremarkable. What is remarkable is the fact that the legislation does not extend to cover all equestrian businesses, but only that of keeping horses for either the purpose of letting them out for hire or for use in giving riding instruction for payment or both, e.g. it does not cover stables which provide only livery. The Acts also place no restrictions on the number of hours which horses may work, though some local authorities restrict the hours by means of a special condition in the licence. There is also pressure for the Act to be amended in respect of both the age of the person left in charge and the qualifications of the licence holder.

The Health and Safety at Work Act 1974

The need for compliance with health and safety legislation has already been discussed in Chapter 3. The 1974 Act (and the regulations made under it) are of great importance. It applies to people, not premises, and covers all employed persons (except domestic employees) wherever they work. Its provisions apply to trainees on government-sponsored training schemes as if they were employees. The Act also applies to those who are not employees in so far as they may be affected by work activities.

The emphasis of the Act is on criminal sanctions and it is enforced on equestrian premises by the local authority which has power to enter premises at any reasonable time or, if there is a dangerous situation, to enter at any time.

Two important weapons available to the local authority are improvement notices and prohibition notices.

- An *improvement notice* can be served where the inspector forms the opinion that someone is contravening a statutory provision and that the contravention is likely to be continued or repeated. It requires the named person to remedy the contravention within a specified period, which must not be less than 21 days.
- A *prohibition notice* can be issued if the inspector thinks that a work activity is being carried on in contravention of statute so as to involve a risk of serious personal injury. It stops the activity being carried on

and can take immediate effect if the inspector forms the opinion that the risk of serious personal injury is imminent, otherwise its operation may be deferred until the end of a specified period. Prohibition orders can be issued on persons, e.g. for a failure to wear prescribed protective clothing.

Appeals against these notices can be made to an industrial tribunal on very limited grounds. Failure to comply with a valid notice is a serious criminal offence.

There is, of course, much other relevant law, but more detailed treatment is outside the scope of this book. If in doubt, you should take competent legal advice.

6 Finance and profit

Raising money

Every business needs capital, and in most cases this means borrowing money. There is no shortage of institutions prepared to lend money, and the method chosen will depend on a variety of factors. The most important of these are size of loan, length of repayment period and the cost.

Mortgages

You can take out a mortgage to buy a business or agricultural property. The mortgage – a charge on the property – is the security for the loan, the amount of which is limited not only by the value of the property but by what you can afford realistically to repay. Mortgage loans are available through the Agricultural Mortgage Corporation or through one of the several mortgage companies. The clearing banks are also willing to consider mortgages. An ordinary building society mortgage is not available for commercial enterprises. In any case, you will need some capital of your own to set up in business, whether this involves buying a property or not. No lender is going to advance 100 per cent of the total purchase price and costs involved.

A comparison should be made on terms – some lenders make a charge for arranging a mortgage and interest rates can vary. Some investors will offer to purchase a property and then lease it back to its former owner who gets the immediate capital injection needed for business purposes but forfeits the opportunity of increasing his capital worth if the property rises in value. Mortgages are for long-term finance; repayment terms of 10 and 20 years are common.

Those who are renting property will need to seek other sources of finance and will have to accept loans which are repayable over a shorter term – usually five years at the most. The most accessible source of finance is the bank where you have your current account; even they will negotiate on terms if really pressed. There are several different types of bank credit, including overdrafts and loans of various sorts which can be used to finance a business. However, you will have to convince the bank manager not only of your creditworthiness but also that the venture is likely to succeed. This means that you must be able to present a good case to him, which in turn involves hard preparatory work.

The bank manager will need to know about you and your commitments and about your knowledge and business experience. Above all, he will need to be be satisfied that your plan is realistic and likely to succeed. You must convince him that there is a market and that you have the knowledge, enthusiasm and ability to succeed.

The bank's primary objective in lending money is to make a profit. The sensible bank manager will insist on seeing a realistic cash flow forecast and budget for at least the forthcoming year. This should show expected receipts and payments (including VAT), private drawings, bank charges and so on. This is certainly essential when embarking on a new venture, but in the case of an established business the audited accounts for the previous years can be used as the basis of your approach. Optimism and enthusiasm are insufficient; the project must be commercially viable.

Overdrafts

Planned overdrafts are one of the cheapest forms of borrowing and are intended for short-term loans. If the bank manager agrees to your request for an overdraft, you will be able to overdraw your current account up to an agreed limit. The amount and the length of the loan is a matter for the bank's discretion – but an overdraft is not meant as a source of long-term finance. A bank manager will usually agree an overdraft facility against a realistic business plan showing clearly when the overdraft will be repaid, e.g. that a horse which is being brought on will be sold in the autumn. Interest is only payable for the period you are actually overdrawn and is between 2 and 5 per cent above the bank's base rate. Interest paid on an overdraft or loan for business purposes may be offset against the business's tax liability.

Ordinary loans

Unlike an overdraft, an ordinary loan must be repaid in regular amounts over an agreed period. The usual maximum is seven years. Typically, interest is only payable on the actual balance outstanding. Security such as an insurance policy may be required for substantial loans. The interest rate is similar to that charged on an overdraft.

Personal loans

The rate of interest on personal loans is fixed at the outset, and the term of the loan is usually two or three years. Personal loans are agreed for a specific purpose and in most cases security is not required although the bank may insist on your taking out life insurance in conjunction with the personal loan so as to ensure its repayment if you die.

Alternatives

Finance houses provide funds for hire purchase or credit sale to enable you to buy a specific piece of equipment or a vehicle. Some finance houses will also provide personal loans, but almost invariably they require security. With hire-purchase, in law you are hiring the goods. They do not become your property until the final instalment is paid. Repayments are normally spread over a maximum period of three years. Hire-purchase is a very expensive form of credit. Instalment repayments also apply where there is a credit sale, but in this case you become the owner of the goods immediately. There is also a form of credit known as 'conditional sale' which is similar to hire-purchase.

Grant aid

The most valuable source of extra capital is grant aid because this does not need to be given back.

Also, grant aid will in some circumstances supplement income for a person starting a new business. Some grants come from the European Union (EU) but most come from the government.

Grants vary from area to area and in some areas grants are very specifically targeted at areas of need. To make the most of grant opportunities it is necessary to consult experts who are up-to-date with current provisions. The two organizations most likely to help a horse business with specialist knowledge of relevant grants are the Agricultural Development and Advisory Service (ADAS) and the Rural Development Commission (formerly CoSIRA); both have regional offices.

Budgeting

A budget is a *plan* of income and expenditure in contrast to accounts, which are a *record* of what has actually happened financially. A budget is a useful financial tool. For example, a buyer wishes to purchase a young horse and bring it on. The buyer has a choice between buying an unbroken horse and having it broken professionally or of buying one that is already broken.

A simple budget of what it will cost to have the horse broken might look like this:

Transport to and from breaking yard	£ 20
Six weeks' livery at £70 per week	£420
Vet, farrier, clipping, etc.	£ 60
Total cost of breaking	£500

On this basis, the buyer can reach a sensible decision provided the estimated costs are accurate.

Similarly, a breeder will need to know when best to sell young stock and the price to ask. A budget can indicate the cost of producing each foal. This might work out as follows:

Depreciation of mare (purchased for £1250; final sale £250 divided by 5 foals)	£ 200
Mare's keep (say 5 foals over 7 years at £400/year)	£ 560
Getting mare in foal	
Stud fee £300	
Livery £150	£ 450
Veterinary expenses	£ 50
Weaning and sale preparation	£ 40
Cost of foal	£1300

If the breeder is an owner-occupier, the value of the property is probably an appreciating asset and so no charge need be made against the foal in the budget. In contrast, if the breeder is a tenant then the cost of (say) 1 ha (2½ acres) would need to be added to the budget costs in order to achieve a realistic figure. This budget does not take account of any labour costs associated with the mare and foal. It also assumes that there is no bank overdraft or other finance charge. If labour costs and bank charges are involved, these will need to be allowed for in the budget. Thus, dependent on the breeder's circumstances, the foal must be sold for between £1700 and £2500 minimum in order to show a gross profit.

To keep the foal on instead of selling it immediately might result in the following pattern, assuming that the foal costs £400 a year for keep:

Foal	£1400
Yearling	£1800
2 year old	£2200
3 year old	£2600
4 year old	£3000

The breeder's dilemma is to decide the point at which the horse may be most profitably sold. In practice, the solution may be to produce the horse under saddle and then sell it; but this increases the risk element in the enterprise. The budget provides some information on which to make a decision.

Another situation arises where the owner of a new livery yard is considering what weekly livery fee to charge. One method of setting the rate would be to consider the charges made by other livery stables in the locality, compare standards and convenience, allow something for breaking into the market, and set the price accordingly. The second way is to prepare a budget and itemise the weekly costs associated with each horse. For example:

Cost of box (rent or maintenance and depreciation)	£ 7
Labour (self + two staff do 15 horses)	£25
Hay (bought from field)	£ 5
Concentrates (based on home-rolled barley)	£ 5
Bedding (shavings to save labour)	£ 5
Stable equipment, electricity and miscellaneous	£ 3
Total weekly cost	£50

To this basic figure, a profit margin must be added so as to produce the weekly charge to clients for each horse at livery.

Budgeting is thus a useful management tool for setting prices, comparing enterprises, making financial decisions and future projections; such budgets are called partial budgets. An overall budget for a project should be comprehensive and have a separate entry for as many items as possible. At the end of the budget period for the enterprise – usually a year – the budget should be compared with what actually happened.

Gross profit contributions

An entrepreneur may be faced with a choice of two enterprises which are equally suited to his holding, and must decide which enterprise is the more viable. One method of doing this is to look at the amount of gross profit produced by each enterprise (called the 'gross profit contribution'), and compare them with a standard. The standard is usually taken to be the average of well-run similar enterprises. The overhead expenses (such as rent, labour, machinery and general expenses) are likely to be the same whichever choice is made, and so they are excluded from the calculations.

The calculation of the gross profit contribution of an enterprise is:

Sales minus *direct costs* = *Gross profit contribution*
(including an allowance
for stock replacement
and extra casual labour)

Agricultural businesses use the very similar concept of the gross margin, which is applied as a management tool in the same way as the gross profit contribution.

Published statistical data on agriculture give average and above average performance figures for different enterprises ranging through the whole spectrum of farming activity. This information is set out in the *Farm Management Pocket Book* which is updated regularly and can be purchased from Wye College, Ashford, Kent TN25 5AH.

When using gross margins or enterprise gross profit figures, it is important to remember that the published standards are only averages based on many holdings in different areas. Although the data is kept up-to-date, local conditions, seasons, market fluctuations and other factors will influence the actual performance of a holding. It must also be remembered that gross profit figures do not represent the 'bottom line' net profit, because the overhead expenses of rent, labour, etc. still need to be deducted. This is done by constructing a partial budget as shown in the following example for putting a new enterprise in place of an old one:

Gross profit for new enterprise	£9,000	
Plus overhead expenses saved	£1,500	
		£10,500
Less:		
Gross profit from old enterprise	£6,000	
Plus extra fixed costs	£2,000	
		−£8,000
Extra net profit		£2,500

Enterprise gross profit contributions are not only useful for planning;

they can also be used to compare actual performance achieved with the performance of similar enterprises elsewhere.

In recent years, many farm incomes have been falling. The situation now in western Europe is that more food is produced than is required. It is too expensive to transport this food to underdeveloped countries and such an expedient can prove to be counter-productive in the long term. It is generally thought best to give underdeveloped countries assistance to make them self-sufficient. Because of the European food surplus, farmers are being encouraged to produce less food, and in order to increase income they are now being forced to look at new enterprises. Forestry is very slow and speciality enterprises such as herbs and venison offer only limited opportunities for a few. Farm gate sales and 'pick-your-own' ventures will continue to be useful, but the likelihood is that a great many farms will turn to the leisure industry. Probably the best hope for farmers lies in a national campaign of 'Riding for All'. The government has offered grants to help farmers establish livery businesses and the restriction on cereals policy will provide more land to ride. Farmers are making efforts to diversify so as to make up the shortfall.

Fortunately, there is now a reference handbook for advisors and all seeking to go into the horse business or improve the efficiency of existing businesses. The *Horse Business Management Reference Handbook* is published by Warwickshire College, Moreton Morrell, Warwick CV35 9BL. It gives figures based on a major national survey updated to reflect current costs and prices. Using the handbook as a reference, a horse business can review its own performance and compare it with other similar enterprises. The comparison will suggest areas for economy and increased output and perhaps enterprises which need discontinuing or radical alteration. It can also be of help in indicating suitable enterprises for exploration.

Facility uptake

Any business must be so managed that it earns its maximum potential, whether it be in terms of staff, stables, horses or any other asset. This is what 'facility uptake' is about. A horse business may have various facilities available, but not all of them may be used to full capacity. The facilities are there, but are not taken up by clients. For example, if a livery yard has twenty boxes, and there is an average of ten horses in the yard at any one time, there is only a facility uptake of 50 per cent. The answer to this problem may lie in cutting the price or, more probably, in better marketing. Again, the working capacity of an instructor teaching five hours daily for five days a week would be 25 hours. However, if the instructor is fully worked for only two days and instructs for only 5 hours in total over the remaining working days, he/she is working at only 40 per cent capacity. The teaching facility and the instructor's capacity is underused. The promotion of mid-week riding could alter the situation. Campaigns can be targeted at housewives and evening rides could be advertised so as to promote a better facility uptake. If evening rides provided the solution, then staff involved would need to be given adequate time off to compensate them for the evening work.

The use of an indoor school provides another example. An indoor school is an expensive capital item and therefore must be used for the maximum number of hours. A local competition horse trainer might be glad to use the school for an hour a day while the resident staff are at lunch. Livery owners might like to have an arrangement to use the school regularly while the staff are having a rest period. A local dog training group might be glad to use the school for one evening, and a local archery group on another. Such users not only provide income by paying for the use of the school, but if vending machines are installed, they will also use them and provide extra income. Moreover, by visiting the establishment regularly for their own purposes, they may well be tempted to ride.

Profitability

Not all equine businesses are profitable. Agriculture again provides some useful lessons because it is also concerned with livestock. An analysis of a group of farms has established that a very small change in either output (productivity) or a reduction in costs will have a large effect on profitability. These minor changes can pass unnoticed until they are forced into focus by a reduction in profit.

For example, for every £100 of costs in the sample group, if average output was £120, but some members received £130 and others only £110, the difference in profitability between these is a variation of the lower group earning only half the average income and the upper group earning 50 per cent more than average. Therefore, for the lower group, an 8 per cent improvement in performance could double the profitability of the business. A small reduction in costs would produce equally dramatic results.

The performance of every aspect of an equestrian business must therefore be scrutinized carefully so as to see if the sales and cost ratios can be increased and decreased. Poor performance – for example, too many mares not in foal on a stud farm or too many ponies at a trekking centre for the number of clients – are easy to spot as indicators of poor management, as are extravagance and wastefulness. An apparently well-managed establishment with excellent performance which is not making an adequate profit may be buying the results at too high a cost. Comparison against standard data and a careful analysis of each enterprise should help to identify this type of problem. The cause may of course be that the total output of the holding is insufficient to meet the owner's needs. If this is the case, the owner must set about increasing output, e.g. by creating new enterprises.

Business management advisors in agriculture – such as those from the Agricultural Development and Advisory Service (ADAS) – are able to use established efficiency measures and have a host of comparative data on which to base comparisons. The horse industry is less fortunate since it has always been secretive about its figures. Modern equine businesses must therefore rely on maintaining good records and making comparisons of performance from year to year against such published data as there is.

A riding school can measure earnings per horse. A stud farm can measure foals weaned against the number of mares owned. As horse people become more conscious of performance details and make comparisons with published data, so management in the industry will become more sophisticated in spotting the strengths and weaknesses of the system.

Economies of scale

Economies of scale can contribute substantially to profitability, and this includes buying in bulk. Bulk buying may involve tying up capital or even obtaining a loan, but nonetheless the saving will justify the costs.

The feed bill is the first area for economy. Barley bought directly from a farmer can be stored in bulk provided it is sufficiently dry. The store must be either a hopper on legs which is filled by a bulk tanker lorry or the store will require a grain auger to carry the feed upwards. In smaller establishments, the alternative is for the grain store to be filled by a bucket. The grain from the bulk store can then be rolled each week to meet the yard's needs.

Feed mills sell mixer rations of high protein food designed to be mixed with barley. Horse feed nuts tend to be very expensive and horses do well on low protein dairy nuts, which are cheaper. Some cattle (beef) nuts contain substances which are poisonous to horses and so care must be taken when choosing nuts.

When purchasing feed direct from merchants, the total quantity of feed can be estimated by type, and quotations for the year's supply can be obtained from competing merchants. Considerable variation will be found in the quotations.

Hay can be purchased direct from the field and is thus handled less often. (The more often fodder is handled, the more it will cost!) Moreover, as winter progresses the price of hay increases. The best possible price is obtained by buying all the hay needed for the season at one time. The safe maxim is 'the larger the quantity, the keener the price'.

Agricultural merchants do not necessarily expect to get the marked price for each item they display when purchases are made in reasonable quantity. Items such as wheelbarrows, buckets, brooms, fencing materials and so on can often be purchased at a discounted price.

Tack shops operate on a mark-up of up to 100 per cent. There is thus some room for negotiation when a tack shop wishes to secure the business of a horse establishment. Even the farrier and the vet are in business and so it is wise to discuss with them what economies can be made so as to keep their accounts at a tolerable level.

The cost of bedding is also worth considering. If straw is used, it costs less from the field. However, wood shavings offer economies in labour and a simple budget will readily show the labour saved against the extra cost of the shavings. If the number of horses and the number of staff remain unchanged, no real saving will be made by changing from straw to shavings, but if an extra horse can be kept with the same staff then a saving is achieved.

Taxation

The first essential for any business is a competent bank manager who can advise on the best sources of finance and help with the financial planning. The second essential is a competent business advisor. The bank manager may double in this role or the advisor may be an independent professional consultant or someone from ADAS or the Rural Development Commission. The third essential is a good accountant. An accountant is not only concerned with auditing but will also ensure that money is not going unnecessarily from the business into the government coffers through the overpayment of tax. The cost of any professional advice is small when compared with the actual and potential savings.

All the advisors should be interested in the business and visit the premises. They should be regarded as friends who are concerned to see the business go from strength to strength. Because grants and taxation change each year, these professionals will keep the business in line with any fiscal opportunities. The owner of the business will certainly need an accountant to advise on and monitor those expenses which can legitimately be offset as business expenses and also to suggest the optimum times for major capital expenditure.

The accountant should advise on and agree to the book-keeping system, since he/she will have to audit the accounts. The simpler and better kept the system is, the quicker (and cheaper) it will be to carry out the annual audit.

The accountant will also be able to give advice about the legal form the business should take – sole trader, partnership or private limited liability company. The principal advantage of a limited liability company is that the liability of the shareholders is limited to the nominal value of the shareholding. If things go wrong the shareholders are not liable to the full extent of their assets if the venture fails because the limited company is a separate legal entity with assets of its own. Another advantage of trading as a limited company is that the owner(s) of the business can become salaried employees of the company as directors. As employees they may be eligible for Social Security benefits (including unemployment pay) if things go wrong. In the case of a sole trader or a partnership, if the business fails and has substantial liabilities, the individual sole trader or partners carry unlimited liability which extends to all personal assets. In the worst case, a sole trader or member of a partnership can be made bankrupt and lose everything, including their home. Insolvency law treats debtors harshly, even if there is no personal fault. However, there may be tax advantages in being self-employed and operating as a sole trader or as a member of a partnership. In every case an accountant's advice should be obtained before deciding on the best sort of business arrangement.

Table 6.1 shows the taxes to be dealt with.

The Inland Revenue compels employers to deduct Schedule E income tax from staff wages each week on the pay as you earn (PAYE) system, together with National Insurance contributions at the appropriate rate. These sums are then sent by the employer to the local income tax office. The Inland Revenue provides employers with the necessary documentation but the system is very complicated and time-consuming. Some people leave the mechanics of PAYE to their accountant; others buy

Table 6.1 Taxation.

---

(1) Income tax
    (a) Personal
        (i) PAYE – for regular employees.
        (ii) Schedule D – for self-employed.
    (b) Business (company) – 'corporation tax'.

(2) Capital tax
    (a) Capital gains tax.
    (b) Inheritance tax (has replaced capital transfer tax).

(3) Value added tax

(4) Special taxes
    (a) Stamp duty.
    (b) Car tax.
    (c) Petrol tax.
    (d) Excise duty on alcohol.

(5) Council tax

---

computer payroll packages which are annually updated.

Taxable income is not the same as gross income, and there are various allowances which are set against the gross income so as to arrive at the taxable income. The Inland Revenue will advise the employer of the employee's individual coding which will take the allowances into account so that income tax is only deductible on earnings above this amount.

Value added tax (VAT) may also have to be contended with. All businesses with a turnover above the prescribed limit must be registered for VAT with the Commissioners of Customs and Excise. As its name suggests, VAT is charged to the customers by the business on its sales and services ('output tax'), and then remitted to the Customs and Excise, usually on a quarterly basis. However, the business is entitled to offset against the output tax the VAT which it has paid on purchases and services ('input tax'). Smaller businesses which operate below the VAT registration limit have an advantage over their VAT-registered competitors when offering livery or other services or selling horses.

One of the advantages of a do-it-yourself (DIY) livery yard is that the clients buy all the necessary feed themselves – usually from the owner of the livery stable – and since animal food is zero rated (i.e. not subject to VAT) the customer saves. Customers may achieve a further saving if, for example, a husband runs a livery business as one entity and his wife runs a feed sale business as another, and the turnover of the livery business is below the VAT level.

Under certain conditions of sale, VAT-registered horse dealers need charge VAT only on their profit and not on the full selling price. This is as a result of the so-called 'second-hand scheme'. The scheme applies to sales from private individuals or from those in business who have sold under the 'margin' scheme. Animals are not eligible if they are being sold for the first time, have been imported by the dealer himself or have been purchased from someone who charged VAT on the full selling price or showed VAT separately on his invoice. Sales must be documented on a special form obtainable for a small charge from the British Equestrian Trade Association (BETA), Wothersome Grange, Bramham, near Wetherby, West Yorkshire LS23 6LY which administers the scheme and from which detailed information can be obtained.

The Agricultural Flat-Rate Scheme (1992) covers the breeding, rearing and care of horses on farms registered and under the Scheme allows these horses to be sold without VAT being charged.

Competitive owners, particularly but not exclusively racehorse owners, are eligible for VAT registration.

Rates

Consideration must be given to the Council Tax. Also it may be advantageous to run an equine business on an agricultural holding although the Rating Officer will differentiate between the two operations. Agricultural buildings are free of the Unified Business Rate but horse buildings are not agricultural, although stud farms can have a concession. The advice of a specialist rating consultant is generally worthwhile and cost effective.

7 Yard management

Routines

Every yard should be so run that there is a happy and relaxed atmosphere in which horses can flourish. It is wisest to have a clear basic daily timetable which is adhered to, although hunting, competitions and other factors may necessitate a change. Horses will readily accept departures from the daily norm provided that there are routines within the timetable.

The timetables in this chapter are based on an eight-hour working day. It is probable that the non-thoroughbred sector will soon follow the thoroughbred sector and other land-based industries so that a basic working week of 40 hours or so will became established. At present, in a great many yards the working week averages between 50 and 60 hours. In modern conditions this cannot really be justified although such owners maintain that the necessary work could not otherwise be done.

The timetables which follow show typical daily routines for three very different types of equine business.

Private, competition or livery yard

07.30 Give small hay feed, check signs of health, check rugs, check empty manger and water.
Muck out.
Give morning feed and leave horses in peace.
08.30 Breakfast. (If staff live out, they may arrive at 08.00 having had breakfast.) Day's exercise list published.
09.00 Quarter all horses, pick out feet into a skip, put on day rugs and bandages (except horses on first exercise). Set fair the yard – everything tidy and in its place.
Tack-up first exercised horses.
09.30 First exercise.

On return, allow the horses to roll and stale.
Groom. (In some yards grooming is done in the afternoon but purists groom after exercise.)
Rug-up.
11.15 Coffee and daily staff meeting.
11.30 Exercise second lot.
12.45 More hay; check water.
Midday feed and leave horses in peace.
13.00 Lunch.
14.00 Exercise third lot.

Note: If grooming was deferred, all three lots of horses will have been exercised during the morning and grooming will be done now. By using a horse walker, or ride and lead, or by lungeing and turning horses out in an exercise paddock, extra horses can be cared for by each member of staff or the time saved to get other essential chores done.

15.30 Clean all tack and drink tea.
16.15 Put on night rugs, skip out, give hay, check water, set fair.
Give evening feed and leave horses in peace.
17.00 Finish (could return from lunch at 14.30 and finish at 17.30).
21.00 Late check and any late feeds

This routine allows for considerable flexibility for the individual horses. The horses requiring the most time will usually be done in the first lot.

Riding school

08.00 Hay, water and feed.
08.15 Some staff muck out. Others fetch ponies from the fields and put them into stalls and groom them.
09.15 Set fair the yard and tack-up for first ride.
Those riding get changed.
09.30 First ride (working pupils).
Exercise livery horses.
10.15 Prepare for second ride. Coffee.

Note: Throughout the day, preparation for each ride starts 15 minutes in advance.

10.30 Second ride (fee-paying students). Other staff do yard chores.
Those on first ride untack, brush off their horses and have coffee.

Note: After each ride all horses are untacked and brushed off throughout the day.

11.30 Third ride. (During term time this could be for 'senior citizens'.) Field and maintenance chores. Exercise remaining livery horses.
12.30 End of morning rides. School hired out.
 Midday stables.
13.00 Lunch.
14.00 Staff return from lunch. (Staff on evening duty have free afternoon.)
14.15 Fourth ride. This might be housewives with small children – provide creche.
15.15 Fifth ride.
 Clean tack and drink tea.
16.15 Sixth ride.
17.15 Feed, hay and water. Put tack in readiness for evening rides.
17.30 High tea. School free for livery owners' use.
18.15 Evening staff on duty.
18.30 Seventh ride.
19.30 Eighth and final ride.
20.30 Night check and evening feeds.
20.45 Lock up.

In this routine all staff take 15 minutes off mid-morning and mid-afternoon and thus also work an eight-hour day.

Racing yard

06.00 Head Lad only feeds and puts up exercise list.
07.00 Lads on yard. Muck out horses in first lot only, brush over, tack-up and tie-up.
 Put in hay and water but leave bed back.
07.45 First lot out for exercise.
09.15 First lot back. Untack, brush over, pick out feet, set bed, rug up. Feed.
09.30 Lads' breakfast.
10.00 Lads on yard. Do second lot.
12.00 Second lot back, done over and fed.
12.30 Half the lads ride out the third lot (the sick, 'lame' and lazy). Remaining lads muck-out their stables and put their feeds ready.

13.15 Third lot back, done over and fed.
13.30 Lads go to lunch and yard is closed.
16.00 Lads return, skip-out and groom horses.
17.00 Trainer's inspection.
         After inspection, each horse is rugged-up, hayed and watered.
17.45 Feed.
18.00 Finish.
21.00 Night check and fourth feed if necessary.

By having extra exercise riders, most of the horses go out on the first two lots but this may mean that several of the lads have to get two horses ready. The day's exercise list shows who will ride each horse at exercise.

Motivation and standards

The first two routines illustrated allow the staff opportunities to use their initiative and skills as thinking riders, teachers and trainers. By giving staff responsibility they will be the more strongly motivated. However, staff should not be left to their own devices without guidance. Inexperienced staff rapidly become demoralized if faced with problems which they do not have the knowledge and experience to solve. The role of management is crucial in setting standards and motivating the team. Guidance, praise, good example and achievable targets stimulate staff to achieve more. The old-fashioned attitude that having paid for a day's work, one can expect a day's work, shows little appreciation of human nature.

Remuneration and benefits

Remuneration is the total reward for service, and includes not only the salary or wage, but the so-called 'fringe benefits' as well. If accommodation is provided, with or without board, staff will appreciate its value if they cost local charges. Board or part board may include use of laundry facilities and so on.

     Riding tuition is also a valuable part of the overall remuneration, but by the same token a lesson missed is the equivalent of a deduction from wages. If employees are to appreciate the value of riding instruction, the lessons must be given as promised; the same applies to instruction in theory and examination practice. Keeping one's own horse at livery as part of the package is fairly easy for someone to cost – but it should be specified in the contract as to whether one can care for one's own horse during working hours. A satisfactory way of dealing with this is to allow the individual to look after his/her own horse but to treat it as any other horse at livery, i.e. the time spent on looking after it is working time which could have been spent on a client's horse.

Allowing staff to use a vehicle for their own purposes can be a valuable perquisite, and it is worthwhile explaining to new staff the running costs involved. Too much must not, however, be made of such things. A safe guide for basic rates is the scale used by the agricultural industry.

Staff working an eight-hour day might have one day off each week and one monthly weekend off. This is the equivalent of a five-and-a-half-hour day or 44-hour working week. Days off in lieu of bank holidays worked must be allowed for, as well as annual paid holidays. The total time off in a year might look like this:

	First year	Subsequent years
Holidays	14 days	20 days
Free weekends	24 days	24 days
In lieu of bank holidays	8 days	8 days
Days off	50 days	50 days
Total days off	96 days	102 days

In fact, allowing for sick leave, possible compassionate leave and days off for training, one might expect each member of staff to work an average of only 260 days in the year. In terms of staff numbers, an example may help: suppose the yard has a fairly level uptake of work throughout the year, and seven staff are needed on duty every day, the calculation to arrive at the staff needed by the business might be:

7 × 365 days = 2555 staff days
2555 staff days/260 days worked = 10 employees

Thus, if seven employees are needed on the yard each day, the business must employ ten people, and a flexible schedule must be worked out to enable each person to go on holiday. A sensible plan is to hold a staff meeting in January of each year to discuss holiday timing, and a year planner can then be displayed in the office to show the holidays and days off of all staff.

Daily duties

Apart from the daily routines, every equine business has days which are different whether because of regular occurrences such as the farrier's visit or a seasonal event like an Open Day. The staff need to know of these things in advance. Wall chart year planners, stocked by most stationers, offer an ideal solution. Self-adhesive labels of differing shapes and colours can be used to denote particular types of activity. Such a planner has already been suggested for staff holidays; a second one can be used to schedule anticipated happenings affecting the yard. Where a year planner is not adequate, then booking boards can be used.

Booking boards

Booking boards are suitable for a busy yard or training stable and for those with many engagements in competitions and so on. Their use and display enables the person answering the telephone to see engagements, deadlines, build-ups to major events and so on.

The recommended system requires two wipe-clean wall boards each permanently marked with a spirit-based pen into a seven column grid for the days of the week, and a cross marked into five columns to allow for the weeks in the month. In use, the first board would be the month of January, and the second the month of February. Information is written onto the grid using an erasable marker, i.e. a water-based pen. At the end of January, all the essential information is copied into a log book as a permanent record. The board is then wiped clean with a damp cloth leaving only the grid, and the month of March is then marked in.

Using this system, there is at least one month ahead clearly on view. But the boards must be sited carefully next to the telephone, and the Head Lad or yard manager must check them each day.

Day work sheets

Pre-prepared day work sheets are a suitable aid to planning. The format will depend on the needs of the business but, once devised, they can be produced quickly and cheaply by any secretarial or printing agency.

Day work sheets can be used to show which horse will be ridden by whom. For example:

Day:		Date:		
Horse	1st lot		2nd lot	3rd lot

In a racing yard, the Head Lad might like to suggest a list, but the trainer checks it and makes the final decisions. The names of the horses in training are filled in in advance and so the trainer needs only to write the rider's name against each horse in one of the three columns. Blanks against a horse's name mean that it is off sick or away racing. The completed day work sheet is posted on the yard notice board first thing every morning.

A similar system used in some racing and schooling yards is based on a magnetic board, and so no writing is involved. Some schooling yards also use a different printed format:

Day:			Date:			
Horse	Start time	Duration	Type of work	Rider	Groom	Special attention

The horses' names can again be written down in advance. This system allows for individuality but is set against the basic daily timetable for the yard.

A riding school is the most complex in terms of a daily work sheet because each horse will work on several occasions. In the case of the suggested timetable, however, lessons are only held eight times. Allowing for a possible indoor school, outdoor school and a hack taking place at any one time, the corresponding daily work sheet could be:

Day:					Date:			
Time:	09.30	10.30	11.30	14.15	15.15	16.15	18.30	19.30
Lesson:	One	Two	Three	Four	Five	Six	Seven	Eight
Instructor:								
Horse:								

If the names of all the horses are written down the left-hand side in advance, overbookings are impossible and the day's work programme is clear immediately. A simple colour code can be used, e.g. red for indoor school, blue for outdoor school, and green for a hack, leaving black for such things as shoeing.

Records

Several questions must be answered if the yard manager is to get the best out of the yard records:

- Why keep the records?
- Who needs to know, when and where?
- Is there a better, quicker, or easier method than the one proposed?
- Where are the appropriate places for the record to be created, stored and used?
- Which method of record-keeping is the most suitable? Card index system, computer or wall boards?

There are some basic records which must be kept by all equine businesses, as discussed in Chapter 4. Other records will depend on the particular enterprise.

A Barn Book should be kept if there is a bulk store from which feed and bedding is transferred to a consumer store on the yard. This method of approach clearly reduces the fire risk in the case of hay and straw. The Barn Book is a simple tally of how much is in the barn.

There should also be a Tack Book in which the tack is listed, and a section for tack which is away at the saddlers for repair or out on loan. It should also have a section for tack which is in stock on a temporary basis, as with a livery horse.

The Vet Book and the Farriery Book mentioned previously will also be kept by the yard manager. The information – including routine attentions such as worming – can be summarized on a wall chart:

Year:

Horse	January	February	etc.
Cassius	Rasp teeth 23 New set of shoes	20 Wormer X 18 Remove shoes	
Jupiter	Rasp teeth 23 Trim feet	7 Vaccination	
etc.			

The number is the day of the month

The wall chart cross-references with the Vet and Farriery Books but presents extra information. It allows trends to be noticed and summaries to be made.

Records for each horse should be kept in a file and should include everything known about the horse and be the place where its Passport or Vaccination Certificate is kept. The file for a livery horse should include a card which is completed when the horse arrives. The livery horse card should include essential information such as the following:

Name of horse   Age   Colour

Owner   Address

Telephone: Daytime
                    Evenings and weekends

Tack delivered:

Other kit delivered:

Condition of horse (including feet, recent scours, etc.):

Some studs and large livery stables like to include a polaroid photograph taken on arrival of the horse held by the person delivering it. The photograph is then attached to the card and establishes identity and visible condition beyond dispute. The file for a livery horse should also include a copy of the livery agreement which should be signed by the owner before the horse is accepted. The agreement will include the terms and conditions for livery, including rate and time of payment and, importantly, should include a clause making the owner responsible for payment of veterinary charges incurred in connection with the horse.

Individual training records may also be kept but these may not be the responsibility of the yard manager. On a stud, stud records will be maintained by the stud groom.

Chores

Many daily chores are ongoing. They include tidying the muck heap, raking the arena, sweeping the yard, washing out feed buckets, checking stock in yard and fields, checking fields, cleaning tack, reporting anything out of order, etc.

The weekly tasks can be apportioned in one of two ways. The first method is to allocate a particular area such as the tack room to one staff member who is then responsible for seeing that it is clean and in good order. The second method is to have a list of chores for each day. The yard manager distributes the tasks and makes the checks at the same time each day. The chores might then be listed as follows:

Monday
: Clean stables, windows, remove cobwebs, etc. Sort out any problems from weekend. Check fields, fences, troughs, etc. Running repairs.
Vehicle check.

Tuesday
: Clean out all drains and drain traps.
Check first aid kits (human and equine) and fire-fighting equipment. Check and replace light bulbs, etc. as necessary. Check all equipment.
Clean out utility room, horse wash area, clipping area, etc.

Wednesday
: Clean out tack room.
Check and clean spare tack. Tack to and from saddler. Clean and disinfect grooming kit. Clean head collars. Do minor repairs to bandages, rugs, etc. Brush out horse rugs.

Thursday
: Clean out feed room and hay/straw barn.
Check feed stocks. Fetch and order feeds.
Scrub out all feed and water vessels not done daily.

Friday
: Clean out office, recreation room, wc, etc.
Check records.
Check shoes. Book farrier.
Level school surfaces, clean gallery, etc.

There are also seasonal chores which are necessary to keep the whole place tidy and in order. It is useful to list these into categories as a reminder of what must be done over the year:

Horse
Dental, worming, tetanus and 'flu injections, lice, etc.
Clipping and trimming.
Roughing off, getting up, fitness.
Competing and/or hunting.
Backing and schooling young horses.
Shoeing and foot trimming.
Rug laundry, tack repairs in closed season, etc.

Stud
Covering, foaling, weaning, culling, sales.

Yard and stables
Roofs and gutters, electrical safety, plumbing.
Spring clean and disinfect, clean out barns.
Painting and pointing.
Maintenance and repairs.
Rodent control, timber preservation.
Checking fire appliances.
Stocking up with hay and straw.

Estate
Fencing – creosote, repair, paint, stone walls, hedges, etc.
Roads, tracks, hard standing.
Gallops, arenas, maneges, cross country, show jumps.
Water troughs, field shelters, hay racks.
Ditches and drains, gates, grids and gateways.
Woodland. Notice boards. Tidiness.
Check transport, MOT, machinery overhaul.
Staff housing and accommodation.

Grassland
Rotational and alternative grazing.
Pick up droppings in paddocks and harrow in fields on hot dry days.
Harrow matted grass. Roll level after winter.
Fertilize, kill weeds, remove poisonous plants, etc., top.

Management
Business appraisal. Records.
Marketing, advertising, public relations, etc.

Planning and budgeting.
Accounts, wages, insurance, taxes, rates, services.
Vehicle licences, etc.
Staff recruitment and training and appraisal.
Buying and selling.
Special events.

Fire

The importance of fire prevention has already been emphasized. It has several important aspects.

Good housekeeping

Litter and waste provide a route for fire. Cupboards should only contain necessary items which should all be neatly stacked and stored. Corridors must be swept daily. Hay and straw should be neatly stacked in the barn, any spillages should be cleaned up and the floor swept regularly. Cobwebs and dust on beams also need regular removal.

Electrics

Unfortunately, both horses and rodents will chew electric cables, and so these are safest in conduits. Adapter plugs should be used with care and precautions should be taken to ensure that they are not overloaded with heavy equipment such as kettles and electric fires. Fuses must never be overloaded. Every electric system for a stable should have an earth trip which cuts everything off if there is a short. If a trip is not fitted, one should be purchased and plugged in before using appliances such as clippers. Great care should be taken when using extension cables. They must always be fully unwound before use and then arranged so that they will not get damaged or cause someone to trip over them. Horses' metal shod feet can cut cables lying on the ground.

Feed and bedding

Damp hay may suffer spontaneous combustion. Hay and straw stores should be positioned so that both stock and people can be safely removed if there is a fire. Fire doors are also very important. The design of any stable complex should allow fires to be isolated and stock removed from either end of any corridor.

Flammable materials

Paint, petrol, bottled gas and similar products must be stored with the greatest care. They should be stored in a separate non-combustible building or shed.

Smoking

Many fires result from carelessness with cigarettes. 'No smoking' notices should be posted, but they must also be obeyed even by the owner and important clients. It is likely that some of the staff will be smokers, and the solution to the problem is to provide an agreed place where smoking is allowed, e.g. the staff room.

Heat

Any heater in the stables should be a permanent fixture and properly fitted. Electric heating is safest for a staff room or a tack room unless there are sufficient offices to justify a central heating system.

Fire-fighting devices

Fire-fighting equipment should be on view in clearly designated spots. It should all be checked regularly and staff must be properly trained in the use of the equipment.

Inspections

A qualified electrician should inspect the electrical system annually to ensure that it is all in safe condition and to combat ongoing wear and tear. The Fire Officer should also look around to spot bad habits, unsafe practices and to check for fire safety.

Fire drill

The fire drill should be outlined clearly on notices with white lettering on a green background. An example might be as overleaf.

   The fire drill needs to be practised within the limits of safety to people and horses. Problems must be identified, e.g. the procedure with a stallion.

FIRE!
SOUND THE ALARM
Alarm button by office door
Handbell and telephone in office – Dial 999
(Emergency key behind glass on wall)
MOVE HORSES IN DANGER
Halters in feed room. Horses to field
Shut both doors of empty stables
TACKLE THE FIRE
only if safe to do so

Work planning

The yard manager needs to spend time with the owner or the business manager to consider the pattern of activities over the year. Different types of yards have different profiles of labour needs. A hunting yard, for example, might calculate that field beans will hold up cubbing until mid-September, the opening meet will be the first Saturday in November, and the final meet will be in mid-March. Each type of yard has its own seasons. In a racing yard there is a set pattern of racing, whilst an eventing yard may get the horses up after their winter lay-off on 2 January each year.

In a stud yard there is a strong pattern of activity. This can be shown as a cyclic diagram in Fig. 7.1.

Work study

Work study is the science of examining the ways of finding the most efficient method of doing a job, especially in terms of time and effort.

In the days when cows were milked by hand, the workers prided themselves on their speed and efficiency. Then milking machines were invented and these were carried down the line in the bier from cow to cow. At this stage, work study came on the scene and devised the milking parlour where the cow not only came to the dairyman and the machine but also stepped up onto a higher level so making work easier. Further study of the time spent on bringing each cow into the parlour led to the herringbone parlour where cows entered and were dealt with in batches.

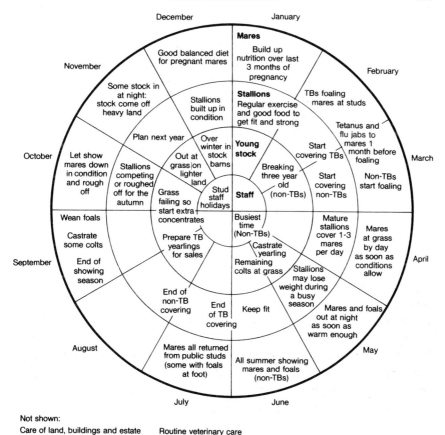

Fig. 7.1 The stud year.

Detailed study led to everything needed being within easy reach; the cowman worked quietly up and down his sunken walkway. The most modern design of milking parlour is the rotary parlour where the cowman stands still and the cows move past on a moving platform.

Similarly, with growing chrysanthemums under glass, originally each plant was staked and ringed and another higher ring was added every few days. As a result of work study, plants are now grown under square meshed pig wire which is stretched tight on four stakes at the corners of the bed. Every few days this mesh is raised a few inches. What was a day's work is now done in a few minutes.

The *Cadre Noir* is the elite and famous display squad of the French cavalry. Their barracks at Saumur are enormous and were recently rebuilt with facilities for hundreds of horses. At feed time, all horses are fed automatically from a central point, the food being conveyed by overhead pipes to each loose box. When mucking out, the men tie up each horse, open the door and then open a trap door to a muck conveyor. The muck is pitched through this trap door and is conveyed away to be deposited on the muck heap which is well clear of the stables.

Every equine business can learn from these examples of work study and modern planning and larger businesses might well benefit from engaging work study consultants.

Flow study/work study

A work study expert will follow a member of staff for a day noting all their movements and then plotting them onto a scale plan of the premises using pins at work points and corners and a piece of thread to mark the person's path. The result of the study may show that the average person working in a stable walks about a great deal. The location of the feed room and the tack room may lead to greater distances being walked than are necessary. Sometimes a door can be cut in a wall to shorten the route and thus save time and effort.

If automatic drinkers have been installed so that staff are no longer needed to carry water and mangers are filled from the outside of each stable, this can save 30 seconds a horse at each feed. With twenty horses this amounts to some four hours a week so that the cost of converting to this system can be covered in less than a year. The time-consuming factor then is the grooms queuing up in the feed room while the head groom hands out the rations for each horse. If all horses can be fed, for example, from four main ingredients plus one of three additives, a simple trolley holding four bins of feed plus a few extra ones could be trundled around the yard, and every horse fed by only one person just as quickly as under the previous system. Even if this resulted in a saving of only two minutes a feed for each of four staff, this amounts to a saving of at least three weeks' work for one person over a period of a year. Similarly, hay racks can have trap doors so that they are filled from the outside. If the hay is fed in wedges and the bale is put on a cart and taken round the stables, the distance travelled by the hay feeder is cut to about one-twentieth and the saving in time is enormous. Time is money.

In some American stables, a section of the wall in the tack room pivots. The required tack is put on this section. The horse is groomed in a stall sited on the other side of the pivoted wall. When the horse is ready, the wall is pivoted and the tack is to hand for tacking up. Untacking works in reverse. In some stables, too, there is a full height cupboard across the

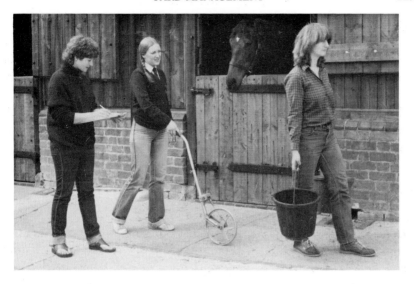

Fig. 7.2 Even simple work study quickly proves how labour-consuming many stable yards are.

corner of every stable holding boots, rugs and grooming kit. Apart from additional hygiene, there is great convenience in having all the correct equipment to hand.

Method study

This is the study of a particular task with a view to improving on the method of doing it. There used to be a pleasant routine called strapping; it was a thorough grooming and body massage for a horse that was expected to perform well on a regular basis. Strapping is still practised in some yards and takes about one hour per horse. If a groom does three horses and straps six days a week, it takes about 18 hours or one-third of the available time. Today, there is generally a shorter working week and horses are groomed less thoroughly and often not strapped at all. If a rotary groomer – with a vacuum attachment to catch the dust – enables a horse to be thoroughly groomed taking 20 minutes less per day and is used on three horses a week, six days a week, this can reduce the working week from the old 54 hours to 48 hours, which is moving towards modern standards. If the six hours of time saved were used elsewhere, it might take eight months to save the cost of the machine.

Road-work with horses is a particularly time-consuming activity. A rotary horse walker can usually take four horses and while the horses are on the walker the staff can be mucking out. This is done more quickly in an empty stable. If four horses on a ride and lead system were out for an hour for each pair and took fifteen minutes a pair to tack up and untack, then the job takes two and a half hours. Using a horse walker, the job can be completed in one hour, including half an hour for mucking out, and thus two hours a day has been saved.

Mucking out is the area of work which lends itself to work study. At the National Stud in Ireland, a tractor and trailer goes round and drops the bales of fresh straw and the muck sheets around the yards. There is one muck sheet for every stable; each sheet has a draw string so that when the stable has been mucked out and the sheet is full it can be pulled tight so as to secure the contents. The tractor and trailer then returns and collects the bundles and takes them to the muck heap. In this method, the use of wheelbarrows is avoided, there is less spilt straw and the job is done more quickly and efficiently. Rubber matting is increasingly being used to reduce the volume of litter and so the labour required. It is also very useful where hygiene is of particular importance. The real breakthrough in bedding for horses is yet to come, but some interesting ideas are under test.

Work study has many specialist areas. Ergonomics, for example, is concerned with the design, comfort and efficiency of the work place. It is also concerned with ideal environments in terms of colour, heat, light and noise. It also studies the design of desks and chairs for those in offices and the key features in any work place.

The more sophisticated work study techniques have little application to the typical stable yard, but many of the basic techniques can be applied so as to get tasks done more efficiently and cost-effectively.

8　Farm and estate

Grassland management

The dairy farmer has a very clear cut attitude towards grass: the more quality grass he can produce, the less concentrates he will have to buy, and fertilizer is cheaper than concentrates. The horsemaster is less clear in his attitudes. He knows that horses do not like lush grass and that their biting mechanism is not suited to long grass. He has no measure of productivity with which to quantify performance, unlike the dairy farmer who can measure the milk produced each day. The regular milk cheque is also a good reminder of the value of grass, whereas horses are only gaining in less tangible factors such as growth and energy. As a result, horse paddocks tend to have little money spent on them, generally have more weeds and less productive species of grass and are only lightly fertilized when compared with dairy grassland. The productivity of grassland and the use made of it depends on many factors. These are shown in Table 8.1.

Table 8.1 Grass production and utilization.

Natural factors	Farming factors	Horse factors
Soil type	Drainage	Worms
Altitude	Acidity	Teeth
Temperature	Sward	Tranquility
Sunlight	Fertilizer	Protection
Rainfall	Management	Safety
Seasonality		
Slope and aspect		
Latitude		

Seasonality

The 'heavier' soils with a higher percentage of clay are more productive but need drainage. The 'lighter' soils with a higher percentage of sand are free draining, low in nutrients and any fertilizer is leached easily away. They also dry out badly in summer but are good to ride on. Within the British Isles, altitude is only occasionally of significance. Temperature affects grass growth. Grass does not grow in the spring until the soil is warm enough and it stops growing in the autumn when the soil gets cooler. South-facing slopes are warmer as they face the sun's rays more directly in spring and autumn. 'Lighter' soils also warm up sooner than the heavier types. The length of the day is a significant factor in determining when the grass starts to grow in the spring; it is later in the north than in the south. Given this mix of natural factors, nature makes every year slightly different and so seasonality alters when growth starts, how growth drops off in mid-summer and when growth stops. These natural factors are beyond human control, but other factors are not.

Drainage is a good example of a factor that can be controlled. Drainage must always be in good order, especially on heavy land. It often starts with a ditch leading to a stream. If the ditch is silted up, the system will not work, and the ditch will need to be cleared out every few years. Along the ditch there will be outfalls where the field drains empty into the ditch: these outfalls must be clear and in good order and above the highest water level in the ditch. If the field drain system is old then it may be necessary to replace it. Signs of the need for drainage include boggy patches, rushes, uneven growth and yellow/green patches. Drainage work is best carried out in summer when the land is drier. Quotations for the work should be obtained from drainage contractors who will advise about grants currently available and queries about grants can be solved by the local ADAS advisor. Mole-ploughing or subsoiling are shorter term forms of drainage; both allow water to move through heavier soil. A drainage contractor can give advice on the suitability of these methods. Both are sometimes included in a new drainage scheme, but generally they must be repeated every few years.

Acidity is the second factor that can be controlled. Soil acidity is measured on a pH scale in which 7 is neutral, below 7 is acid, and over 7 is alkaline. Grass grows perfectly well in slightly acid conditions such as a pH of 6, but below that production will fall. If the soil is too acid, the wrong plants will prosper. The remedy for acidity is chalk or lime, and a competent contractor will use the material most economically available in the area. Contractors will test the fields to see if lime is needed. It is bad practice to over-lime because an alkaline soil does not so easily provide minerals necessary for the growth and health of the crop. The frequency of liming depends on soil type, but every eight years or so is average.

A third factor needing attention is the composition of the sward. Generally, a grass sward is made up of different grass species together with some clovers and herbs. A new ley will have a carefully selected range of high-yielding varieties of a few selected species. The most productive grass in Britain is perennial ryegrass and generally this should form the majority of the sward. Horses like tall fescue, so a little may be included. Because horses gallop about and thus punish the sward, it is a good plan to include some creeping type of grass such as creeping red fescue so as to give the sward a good bottom. A little wild white clover will provide some nitrogen to assist the grasses. Seed mixtures are discussed in greater detail in *Pasture Management for Horses and Ponies* by Gillian McCarthy (Blackwell Science).

A ley is a planted grass crop as opposed to permanent pasture. On farms, there are short term leys of one or two years duration and longer leys of five to eight years. After that length of time a ley will have deteriorated into less productive grasses and weed grasses and so will need re-establishing. On most horse establishments this will be done by contractors using sod seeders. A field which has got worn or thin in patches can be refurbished by rough harrowing, followed by broadcasting seed and fertilizer and then rolling. This work must be carried out in the spring or when it is warm and there is sufficient moisture in the soil.

Food for the grass is the fourth factor. Plants, like animals, need food to survive and need plenty of food if they are to grow well. Soil contains natural plant foods, but fertilizer must be added for extra growth. Farmyard manure was the original form of fertilizer. Horse manure is not generally used for horse paddocks as its use would spread worm eggs. There are some other organic fertilizers but they tend to be expensive. Some horse owners prefer them because they release their nutrients more slowly and contain trace elements.

Most people use inorganic fertilizers. These are usually compounded into each granule or are mixed; the latter are cheaper but possibly not quite so efficient. A possible compromise for horse paddocks is to use semi-organic fertilizers and these may be particularly suitable for studs. For mature horses, a typical programme would be to use inorganic fertilizer with an analysis of 25 per cent nitrogen (N), 10 per cent phosphate (P_2O_5) and 10 per cent potash (K_2) at a rate of two 50 kg bags per acre in the spring and a top dressing of one bag of straight nitrogen fertilizer (34.5 per cent N) after each grazing. A compound with a little extra potash may be given after a hay cut so as to make up for the nutrients carted off the field with the crop. Grazing stock return many of the nutrients to the soil. It is normal to keep stock off the newly fertilized field until a shower of rain has washed the fertilizer into the ground.

Good management greatly affects the yield of grass. The aim is to graze down the grass, without eating the heart out of it, and then to give it a good rest while it recovers and regrows. An ideal system would be a group of compatible horses, as at a riding school, which can all graze together. The horses are rotated around, say, five paddocks (Fig. 8.1). After each grazing by the horses, sheep or cattle graze to clean up the paddock and dispose of some of the worms. Cattle will also eat off long grass. An alternative is to top the paddock at this stage. The important point is that grasses and weeds rejected by the horses must not grow on and seed or they will increase and the paddock will deteriorate. The paddock is then top dressed with a small amount of nitrogen fertilizer. Then it is rested.

The nature of grass growth is such that it peaks in late spring and has a mini-peak in the early autumn. The spring peak can be taken for hay or silage and the autumn peak allows a field to be shut up and used later as 'hay on the stalk' or foggage (dead grass grazed in situ). The system of paddocks allows for a different paddock to be used for conservation each year. The paddock used for the winter should be the best drained one. It will get badly poached but it is important to concentrate this damage and not to spread it across all the fields. In a larger field where there is no paddock system, grazing of new grass can be controlled using electric horse fences which have broad orange, yellow or silver tapes. These fences can also be used to provide a wider barrier between fields where it is necessary to prevent horses sniffing at each other over the fence. Care must be taken with electric fences near water troughs.

Grassland needs little attention apart from topping. At the end of the winter, the paddocks can be chain harrowed to tear away the old dead and matted grass and open up the sward. The grass may then be rolled to encourage tillering (production of new shoots), to reduce any winter 'puffiness' in the soil and to level out the effects of poaching. The timing of this rolling is crucial on some soils. Paddocks can be harrowed on dry hot days so as to scatter dung which is then desiccated by the sun and wind. To do this on warm wet days would spread worm eggs which flourish in such conditions. On small fields droppings can be collected either by hand or by a special field-type tractor-mounted vacuum cleaner as an aid to worm control.

Weeds will be largely controlled by regular topping, but it may be necessary to use herbicides occasionally. Current statutory regulations

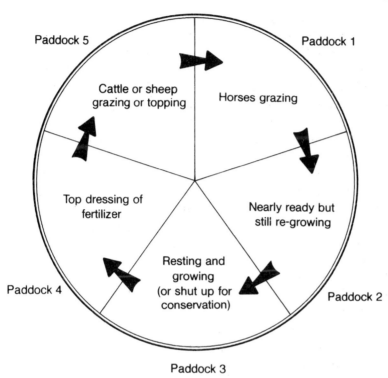

The activities rotate round the paddocks

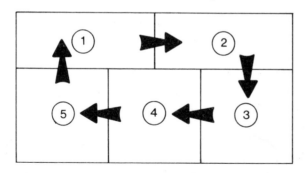

Fig. 8.1 Rotation of paddocks.

provide that staff may not be asked to use herbicides unless they have been specifically trained and so it may be necessary to call in a contractor. Good work can be done by hand as in pulling ragwort, clearing woody nightshade from the hedges and topping awkward corners with a strimmer. Banks and boundaries are often wild areas which act as a source of weed infestation to the fields, and weeds (especially docks and thistles) should be cut down in those areas before they seed.

The horse factors which ensure the best use of grassland include regular worm treatment and an annual check on the horses' teeth for the removal of sharp edges. Tranquillity is important to horses and although they soon get used to fields by busy roads or railway lines, they find it worrying to be the occasional source of amusement to marauding children from housing estates. Protection must be provided and the preferred type is a good hedge which has been allowed to overgrow. The protection is from sun and flies in the summer and wind and rain in the winter. Banks, buildings and trees (protected from having their bark chewed) all provide shelter.

Windbreaks can be made using plastic windbreak set on strong wooden frames. Windbreaks can be set round two sides of the field corner or in an open space in a Y formation to provide protection from all angles. A field shelter should not have one central entrance if several horses may use it, as bullying can occur within. Excellent buildings for over-wintering in the fields are those which provide both a shelter for horses and a store for the hay, with the hay racks being under cover. Further protection for horse fields is provided by planting trees in small circular groups in the field or in plantations set in rounded-off corners. Some local authorities will provide trees free of charge for such purposes. Also grants are available for tree and hedge planting; the Farming and Wildlife Advisory Group field officer for the county can advise on these.

All fences should be safe, tidy, smart, stand up to pressure, not need painting, not get chewed and be inexpensive. With timber fences, a single strained wire set one inch above the top rail will prevent chewing. A lower electric wire will stop cattle from pushing against the fence and discourage horses from rubbing. An alternative top is a white strip which is tensioned on two wires; such modern materials can be erected more quickly and thus save on labour costs. Mesh at low level will control sheep but it can also catch horses' feet particularly if it is a single dividing fence. Mesh is therefore best used only for the perimeter fence. If trees are set in a double fence between fields, it is well to reckon on a horse reaching two metres to try and bite the young shoots. To make the gateways safe in winter it is a good plan to build up the area round both sides of a gateway for an overwintering field. The procedure is to lay a builder's permeable membrane and tip on to it material which will settle to a firm surface, such as stone topped with grit. Transport is a high proportion of the cost of the material used. Similar treatment can be given to the areas around field shelters and water troughs.

A final aspect of paddock safety is the control of poisonous plants. Many mildly poisonous plants will not be eaten by horses unless they are very short of food, so privet, box, rhododendron and laurel in hedges are not ideal but are not generally a problem. However, hedge clippings of any of these could lead to trouble if tipped in the field.

Acorns are poisonous if eaten in large quantities and so oak trees can be a seasonal problem. Horses do not generally eat broom, but it is poisonous and should be avoided. Yew can be fatal, even in small quantities. Laburnum is poisonous, especially the seeds. In the hedges, woody nightshade is poisonous, while both black and white bryony has poisons in the roots if chewed. Old man's beard is also poisonous but it does not seem to tempt horses.

In the field, ragwort must not go into the hay and although horses normally avoid mature plants, they might nibble young growth and it is a cumulative poison. Wild arum or cuckoo pint (Lords and Ladies) may be found under the hedge: it has bright red poisonous berries. Buttercups are not good for horses although poisoning is rare. Bracken has poisonous roots and the leaves are bad for horses, although it is usually rejected. Foxgloves and horsetails are also poisonous and must not be included in the hay. Other poisonous plants include dog's mercury, water and spotted hemlock, water dropwort, deadly and black nightshade, lupins, meadow saffron, purple milk vetch, St John's wort, thorn apple and charlock. Many toadstools are also poisonous.

Conservation

Because the production of grass is uneven through the seasons (Fig. 8.2) there is likely to be spare grass in spring which can be allowed to grow on and be cut as hay or silage for use in winter. Ideally, hay should be cut at

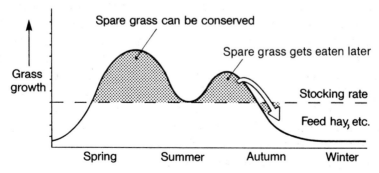

Fig. 8.2 Grass production. The graph shows how the growth of grass varies with the seasons.

the flowering stage before it goes to seed. If it is cut sooner the yield will be less; if cut later, the quality will be greatly reduced. The major problem with making hay in Britain is that a week of fine weather is needed. The hay needs regular spreading and turning and putting up into rows if rain threatens. It is no good relying on a contractor for these operations and suitable implements must be purchased. Mowing the hay can be done by a contractor unless the topping mower is also suitable for heavy stands of long grass. Baling the hay is another problem, as a contractor will tend to concentrate on bigger clients, and the purchase of a good second-hand baler may provide the answer. The alternative is to put the hay on tripods by hand as is still done in parts of Europe other than Great Britain. The practical problems may be avoided if the hay is sold as it stands.

Silage is an alternative to hay. The principle of silage making is that grass without air will pickle in its own juices by partial fermentation. Tower silage is very expensive in terms of capital outlay. Clamp silage is excellent but presents feeding problems for horses. The usual procedure is to cut out the amount needed each day and take it to the horses although some people have successfully allowed the horses to feed direct from the face of the silage clamp.

At least two major horse establishments claim that going over to silage from hay was the single most significant improvement in their profitability. Clamp silage can be made by a local farmer or contractor. It can be made by mowing, wilting and carting with a buckrake, but it is better made with a forage harvester which picks up from the wilted sward and chops the grass before blowing it into a high-sided trailer for transport to the clamp. Alternatively, the wilted sward may be made into big round bales which are then sealed in black polythene, but this again calls for contractor's equipment.

Problems can arise if dirt is allowed to contaminate the silage and give rise to toxic material. The bales are also rather variable in quality, and a big bale is difficult to handle. There must be sufficient stock to enable a big bale to be cut up and used within a few days. If silage is being introduced as a new food, it will be found that the horses are not very keen for the first week or so and will lose a little condition. However, they will soon put it back on and should be well settled to the new diet within a fortnight.

Complementary farming

Beef, sheep and hay for sale are common enterprises on horse establishments. Analysis of profitability figures shows that there is no easy way to supplement the income from horses. The profitability of livestock has generally decreased in recent years and intensive livestock needs a high degree of skill and experience to achieve satisfactory returns. However, it is often appropriate for the horse business to have some complementary farm enterprises so as to optimize on the resources of the holding, just as many farmers have turned to alternative enterprises ranging from providing bed and breakfast accommodation to more exotic pursuits such as hang-gliding (Table 8.2).

Table 8.2 Results of a survey of eight central southern counties showing the various alternative enterprises in action on farms.

Adventure and war games	Herbs
Angora goats	Hunting
Bee farming	Mail order
Cakes	Meat
Cheese	Metalwork
Cider	Mills
Clothes	Mohair
Cottages	Quails
Craft shops	Shooting
Farm museum	Snails
Farm shops	Water gardens
Fish – trout and ornamental	Water skiing and sailing
Food storage	Wine
Goats milk	Wood
Gun dogs	Wood furniture
Hang-gliding	

Sheep

The value of sheep as grazers complementary to horses is well established. With good management, each ewe will produce a fleece and two lambs which fatten on grass and this produces an acceptable profit. Sheep need good fencing as they are notorious for getting out. If the land is very wet, sheep are best over-wintered in a barn and can be lambed indoors or out. Any lambing area which is used again the following year creates an increased risk of disease and so extra care must be taken if lambing indoors. Fat lamb prices are least from July to November. They are highest at Easter, but it takes specialist skill to alter the natural season of production. There are enterprises where sheep are shorn twice a year, but in practice it may be difficult to find anyone willing to shear a very small flock as the setting-up time may be out of proportion to the shearing time.

Sheep milk production is a newly popular enterprise. An East Friesland ewe can produce 200 gallons of milk a year. Modern sheep milking parlours are easy to use. The milk has a good retail sale value and can also be made into cheese.

All sheep need dipping. Small individual dips are available or else the flock can be taken to a neighbour's sheep dip. This is to the advantage of both parties as the more sheep using the dip, the less it costs for each beast.

Multiple suckling cows at grass

Multiple suckling cows provide a good return on the land grazed. The system is that a cow has extra calves put to suckle her, the calves being bought at market when they are a week old. Four calves to a cow is the usual number as they can suckle simultaneously, although a high-yielding cow may take two more calves. Calf mortality can be expected at 5 to 10 per cent – the higher number if there are more calves on each cow. There are problems likely with any young stock, but the system offers a good monetary return for those who are able to cope.

Beef

A few beef cattle can be bought at market to graze behind the horses. Cattle need strong fencing. When the animals are no longer required in the autumn, they can be resold at market. They should have put on weight steadily and will thus provide a small profit. If cattle are to be over-wintered, there must be suitable buildings available and a great deal of feed will be consumed. In recent years, profits have been very variable, even for those with considerable experience.

Bucket rearing of early weaned calves

Newly weaned calves are either bought at one week old in the market or obtained under a rearing contract with a farmer or local co-operative. The calves need fresh air without draughts, and in the first three weeks one calf in thirty may die. They feed on milk substitute up to the age of five weeks, but gradually settle onto weaner pellets and then go on to rearer nuts and hay. The calves are bedded on straw and kept in small groups. It is a false economy to keep them short on food because their value at the age of six months is dependent on how well they have done.

Attention to detail, hygiene, good stockmanship and experience all help to raise performance.

Veal production

Strong Friesian bull calves are purchased at a week old. They were sometimes reared in individual pens, but excellent results have been obtained by loose-housing the calves in groups. Profitability depends on buying the calves at a reasonable price, achieving a high food conversion ratio, low mortality rate and a good price at the end. A 45 kg calf will grow to about 170 kg in fifteen weeks, resulting in a dressed carcase of 100 kg.

Pigs

Pigs are an unsuitable enterprise except for the specialist because of modern demands of scale and efficiency. The market tends to be cyclical and horses do not like pigs. However, for those who like pigs or appreciate the special flavour of home-reared pork one or two 'backyard pigs' can be fattened without a great deal of trouble.

Egg production

Where hens are battery housed there is a considerable capital outlay in terms of cages, buildings and feed hoppers. A high degree of efficiency is needed because the profit margin per egg is so small. The birds are bought at point-of-lay, and after a year they are worn out and fetch little if sold.

Free range poultry may have more appeal and can be profitable if there is a good yard gate sale potential. Foxes are a particular hazard. Their cunning and ingenuity should not be underestimated nor should the devastation they can cause on the one night the hen house is not properly closed. At the end of their productive life, the hens, plucked and dressed, will also have a reasonable yard gate sale value.

Table poultry production

Broiler production is another of the finely balanced intensive livestock enterprises, and many smaller producers have found that they cannot compete with the bigger operators. The same is now true of turkeys, and even at Christmas they show little return for the labour. Table ducklings fattened in eight weeks are also less viable than they were, but provided they are well-managed and the mortality rate is low they can still be worthwhile.

Rabbit meat production

The usual way to get involved is as a contract producer for a large rabbit meat marketing company. The necessary equipment includes buildings and cages and the buying company will advise on source of stock and technical matters. The food conversion rate is critical and so it is essential to use a well-tried specialist feed. The does are prolific, mating is easy and technical problems are generally infrequent. The rabbits are sold alive and show a modest profit if treated as a sideline.

Other crops

Fruit orchards can be profitable but are a long-term investment. Foreign competition has depressed the profits of British orchards.

Forestry is an even longer term investment and is not for those with limited acreage. Its profits depend on grants and/or taxation advantages. Fast-growing timber cropped regularly for burning (called biomass) may be practicable, and growing Christmas trees is another possibility. For further information see Richards *et al.*: *Trees as a Farm Crop* (Blackwell Science).

All forms of horticulture require specialist knowledge, training and experience and so while field-scale vegetables or a garden centre could be complementary enterprises to a horse business, a specialist partner or manager would be needed.

Three enterprises have been found to be particularly good complementary ones:

- *'Pick your own' vegetables or soft fruit.* This could share parking, toilet and refreshment facilities with a riding school.
- *Herbs.* The increasing interest in herbs has given rise to many successful herb farms. Specialist growing expertise is needed, but a herb farm can also utilize relatively unskilled labour in packing. This can provide evening work and extra money for staff.
- *Mushrooms.* Mushroom growing is a useful enterprise and can provide an income in units which can be increased to suit need. However, it is not an easy option. Horse manure needs to be sterilized and then mixed with chalk as the growing medium and this requires specialist equipment. Mushroom growers are also suffering intense competition from overseas growers.

Estate maintenance

It is essential that the manager takes careful stock of the capital asset represented by the property itself. Land and buildings are valuable and generally appreciate ahead of inflation and in response to the scarcity of suitable equestrian properties.

Choice of colour in paintwork, the planting of trees and shrubs and the choice and materials and siting of new buildings are all matters which will affect a visitor's first impressions of the property. First impressions will influence every potential client and also affect the price if the property is put up for sale. The plan should therefore be to create the right ambience and an impression which is welcoming, smart and in good taste. Every time something needs repairing or repainting, an opportunity is presented to move in the right direction. The overall design should have been thought through carefully, even though it may take many years to achieve the desired result. Phased expenditure over and above the basic maintenance costs usually proves a wise investment.

When repairing buildings or facilities, consideration must be given to their economic use and the justifiable expenditure. How the repair should be carried out economically and efficiently and using modern methods and materials is also important. The method used will always be influenced by the building's original construction. All materials used must be strong and durable as horses and the British climate combine to create heavy wear and tear. A temporary expedient is a false economy because it means that the job has to be done twice and almost inevitably the final repair is put off, often for years. Although the owners may get used to the look of the 'patched up' job, customers may regard it as an eyesore and infer that the horse care is of the same standard.

It is sensible to keep an Estate Book in which any property damage and necessary repairs are noted by staff so that when suitable staff or contractors are available there is a record of what needs to be done. There should also be an annual plan for the routine estate jobs – fencing, painting, pointing and so on. If planned new facilities and building works are added, one creates a properly phased maintenance and construction plan.

If major works are required, quotations will be obtained from outside contractors. The common practice is to seek estimates from three tenderers, and if the work is substantial it is sensible to prepare a written specification showing exactly what is required. Most building contractors will submit estimates incorporating their own conditions although for larger projects standard national contract conditions are available and the work will be carried out under an architect's supervision. Obviously common sense must be used: the local jobbing builder with a good reputation may not have the office resources to prepare detailed estimates, but many lawyers' fortunes have been made from building contract disputes, particularly where a firm price has not been agreed.

Fences, ditches, roadways, paths and all other physical aspects of the estate must also be cared for. Machinery also needs carefully planned servicing in line with the manufacturer's recommendations. These things are all too often neglected, but a squeaking wheel on a wheelbarrow or an under-inflated tyre are signs of bad management, just as a decrepit building is.

9   Enterprises

Introduction

A horse business often consists of several equine enterprises and it is rare to find that a particular business is completely self-sufficient. Many riding schools, for example, combine the giving of riding instruction with taking horses at livery and a certain amount of dealing. Trekking centres commonly provide full board accommodation as well. Table 9.1 provides a checklist, and some of the more important enterprises are discussed in this chapter.

Table 9.1 Checklist of equestrian enterprises.

(1) Livery stables.
(2) Dealing – buying, selling, advising.
(3) Riding lessons – possibly for lessons leading to exams.
(4) Hirelings – possibly for lessons, hacking, trekking, hunting, competitions, etc.
(5) Training – horse and rider combinations for competitions.
(6) Driving – for pleasure, for exams, for functions.
(7) Equestrian services – use of school, jumps, cross-country, gallops, hire of dressage arenas, show jumps, clipping, etc.
(8) Managing agent for YT or other government schemes.
(9) Running horse shows on own premises or for others.
(10) Stud farm – breeding horses, stallions at stud, mares at livery, rearing young stock, training staff for exams.
(11) Lecturing, demonstrations, training days, clinics, etc.
(12) Accommodation for clients.
(13) Resident farrier.
(14) Consultancy.
(15) Country club and/or equestrian club.
(16) Rehabilitation centre, performance development, vet centre.
(17) Time-share horses.

Livery

A livery yard is one where other people's horses are cared for and stabled in return for a fee. Although the Riding Establishments Acts do not at present cover livery yards, the premises should be at least up to the statutory standards, i.e. that the accommodation for horses is 'suitable as respects construction, size, number of occupants, lighting, ventilation, drainage and cleanliness'. Grazing offered should be maintained in good condition and fields should never be overcrowded. All horses on the premises should be well cared for. The premises should be kept hygienic and safe, and there must be proper provision for horse food, bedding and tack. There should be adequate fire precautions and fire prevention equipment so as to prevent fires and safeguard both people and horses.

There are various types of livery:

- *Full livery*. This offers full care of the animal in return for payment.
- *Schooling/stud/hunting livery*. This offers full care together with breaking, schooling, hunting or whatever else is contracted for.
- *Part livery*. This is also known as half livery or working livery and is where care of the horse is offered in return for its use by the operator as full or part payment. Establishments offering this service must normally be licensed by the local authority under the Riding Establishments Acts.
- *Grass livery*. This is the provision of supervised grazing and perhaps shelter. Any provision for supplementary feeding must be specified and agreed.
- *Do-it-yourself livery*, where only facilities are provided in return for payment. Under this arrangement, feeding, care and exercise is the responsibility of the animal's owner.

It is sensible for the livery contract to be in writing, and the British Horse Society has published valuable guidelines as to what a livery contract should contain. All livery contracts should contain:

- names of the parties;
- type of livery, weekly rate, method of billing, any additional extras provided, and daily terms of the contract;
- names of veterinary surgeon(s) and registered farrier to be used;
- responsibility for insurance;
- responsibility for innoculation against tetanus and 'flu;
- any stable rules, e.g. wearing of BSI-approved hard hats, riding

restrictions, parking areas, notice required to move the horse out of hours;
- emergency contacts;
- notice required for terminating contract on either side.

Other provisions must be made additionally in contracts for livery of different sorts and these are shown in Table 9.2. In all cases, the ultimate responsibility for the care of the horse rests with the owner or operator of the livery yard while the horse is in his/her charge.

A livery stable needs a set of rules and general procedures if it is to operate pleasantly and efficiently and many of the points made in the specimen set of DIY livery rules set out below are applicable to other types of livery. Transport is sometimes a problem with hunting livery and

Table 9.2 Contents of a contract for livery, depending on type.

	Full	DIY	Grass	Working
Watering and feeding	•	•	•	•
Turning out and checking		•		
Vaccination, worming and teeth	•	•	•	•
Farriery	•	•	•	•
Stabling and bedding		•		
Forage and concentrates		•		
Mucking out		•		
Grooming	•	•		•
Security		•		
Tack cleaning	•	•		•
Emergency call outs (vet, etc.)	•	•	•	•
Checking on horse			•	
Security of fences			•	
Access to paddocks		•	•	
Care of box and bedding	•			•
Exercise	•			•
Hours of work: day/week				•
Types of work				•
Types of rider: skill/weight				•
Access to exercise areas	•	•	•	•
Use of facilities	•	•	•	•

Specialist liveries such as hunting, point-to-pointers, show horses and ponies and so on will need considerable extra detail concerning these activities in the contract.

if the operator is offering a transport service on hunting days this may affect the position of both road licence and insurance.

The most difficult service to operate is undoubtedly a DIY livery if only because the operator has the least control of the situation. If standards are to be maintained a clear set of rules must be strictly enforced.

Specimen rules for a DIY livery yard

These rules should be agreed and signed by the owner of the horse before the animal is accepted in the yard, and are best incorporated as an annexe to the formal livery contract. 'Horses' in these rules includes ponies.

(1) All horses must be cared for in accordance with the standards specified in s. (4)(b) of the Riding Establishments Act 1964.
(2) Any owner who fails to keep his/her horse to the required standard or who behaves in a manner which is detrimental to the other owners or the operation of these stables will be required to take their horse(s) elsewhere if they persist in such conduct after due warning.
(3) Owners are fully responsible for any damage to persons or property caused by or in connection with their horses and must have at least third-party liability insurance.
(4) The operator reserves the right to call in a veterinary surgeon to a horse at any time and the horse's owner agrees to be fully responsible for any costs so incurred.
(5) All horses must be innoculated against tetanus and equine 'flu and the owner must maintain up-to-date records showing such innoculations.
(6) All horses must be wormed to the following programme [which should be specified].
(7) The feet of all horses shall be properly cared for.
(8) No smoking is allowed on the premises.
(9) Properly fitting and secured hats in good condition and conforming to current BSI specifications must be worn on horseback at all times.
(10) Suitable footwear with well defined heels must be worn when riding.
(11) The doors and gates of all riding areas must be closed before riding commences.
(12) No riding is allowed among grazing horses.
(13) All tack and equipment must be labelled with the owner's name or identifying mark and must be kept in the tack room which must be locked after use. [Each individual should have an individual small tack/feed room, otherwise disputes are inevitable.]

(14) No person is allowed on the yard before 07.00 or after 20.00 except with the prior permission of the proprietor.

(15) All horses must be cared for in accordance with the following timetable:

> Mucked out and fed by 09.00.
> At least 20 minutes exercise must be given daily.
> Groomed (including picking out the feet) every day.
> Evening feed between 16.30 and 19.00.

(16) The following services are available on request. In all cases where owners fail to comply with Rule 15 the relevant services will be provided and charged for by the proprietor:

Concentrate feed (including food)	£1
Hay per feed	£1
Mucking out	£1
Bale of straw	£1
20 minutes exercise on horse-walker	£1
Grooming	£1
Horse holding for vet/farrier as needed	£3 per hour
Full care of pony (up to 14.2 hands)	£5 per day
	£30 per week
Full care of horse (over 14.2 hands)	£7 per day
	£40 per week
Schooling (40 to 60 minutes)	£5 to £15 depending on rider agreed
Road exercise (ride and lead)	£3 per hour
Lesson (about 45 minutes)	£10 to £20 each according to instructor and number of pupils
Clipping	£10 to £20 according to size and clip
Trimming and plaiting	£5 mane or tail
Hire of pony-size loose box	£15 weekly
Hire of loose box (horse size)	£17 weekly
Hire of individual tack/feed room	£5 weekly
Trailer parking	£5 weekly
Horsebox parking	£7 weekly
Use of riding field	FREE
Use of outdoor school	£1 per horse/session
Use of indoor school	£2 per horse/session

Use of lights	£1 per horse/session
*Use of jumps	£2 per horse/session
*Use of cross-country course	£5 per horse/session

N.B. Asterisked items must be booked in advance.

Please note that bedding, hay, feed and equipment can be purchased on the premises at the following times: [specify].

Farmers intending to take advantage of grants available to diversify their activities by going into the livery business must consider the possible need for planning permission for a change of use, as well as the likely effect on rates. The regulations about grants and related matters are changed constantly and advice on the current position should be obtained from ADAS.

Dealing

At one time horse dealers had the bad reputation now reserved for dealers in low-priced second-hand motor vehicles. Horse dealers are now fewer and more widely scattered and rely on their good reputation. A dissatisfied customer is generally bad news to a dealer who will try and replace a horse which does not suit a client. However, clients can ruin good horses very quickly and bad riders tend to blame the horse for their lack of success. Horses are also rather prone to problems.

A horse dealer needs to be a rapid and good judge of both horse and customer as well as a good negotiator. Some clients expect to pay the price being asked and will go home rather than haggle if the initial asking price is too high. Others will enjoy bargaining and may well appreciate liquid refreshment while doing so.

Clients start making judgements about standards and quality as soon as they enter the premises. They continue to make judgements when they meet the dealer and as they observe the standards of stable management. However under-capitalized the business may in fact be, its standards must be of the highest. An extra bale of straw and well-banked sides suggest a real horse-person with good old-fashioned values and attention to detail. Clean but well-worn working gear, being ready on time and remembering the client's name all help to conclude the sale. One well-known dealer keeps a card file of customers and makes a note of the names of the client's spouse and children. This attention to detail both surprises and reassures a client if he/she returns some years later.

When a horse is presented, there must be a good place to stand it. If the horse is extra tall, the customer should look slightly down on it. If the horse is a little smaller than required, the horse should be on ground which is imperceptibly higher than the customer. The dealer must select the horse's best side and angle with care – the early moments are important.

When the horse is shown in hand, there must be a suitable hard level strip on which the horse can be shown to advantage. The horse should be tacked-up by staff so that the dealer can concentrate on the client. If it seems likely that another horse in the yard might be suitable for the client, staff must be forewarned. One performance horse dealer stands with his clients in the indoor school and calls up each horse on a CB radio, with a team of staff bringing horses, demonstrating them over the jumps and taking them away. Another dealer shows his clients two or three horses, has them try them and then takes the client to his office where comfortable chairs, a fire and a drinks cupboard help to create the right atmosphere for buying.

The client must expect to pay for the dealer's experience and expertise. Buying a horse from a friend is a good way to lose a friend. To buy from a sale is often to buy untried. Buying from a dealer is often best and safest. A dealer will generally try to turn his/her stock over fairly quickly because it costs over £50 a week to keep a horse and the price the dealer has paid is capital tied up. A dealer with a yard of ten boxes will probably need £400 a week to run the yard. If the dealer has a mortgage on the property and is operating on borrowed capital, he/she may well need £70 a week to service the borrowings. He/she probably needs a further £100 a week to run a house, a car to view the horses and a lorry to collect them. If one deal in ten ends up unprofitable and the dealer sells an average of two horses a week, he/she will need to add £300 to each horse over the amount it cost to acquire. On top of this, he/she needs to add profit (say £150) and to allow a negotiating margin he/she adds a further £150. So if the dealer buys a horse for £2,000 and its vetting cost £50, plus a further £50 for a horse that failed the vet, the dealer must put the horse on the market at £2,700. If the same dealer sells only one horse a week, then his £2,000 purchase must be put on the market at £3,250. This example illustrates the need for a dealer to achieve volume and fast turnover if he/she is to make a regular living from dealing.

Riding schools

A riding school must have planning permission to operate as well as a

Riding Establishment licence. To obtain the licence the applicant must, among other things, hold a current insurance policy which insures him/her against liability for any injury sustained by those who hire a horse for riding and those who use a horse in the course of receiving riding instruction from him/her in return for payment, as well as covering third party liability. Employers' liability insurance will also be required and desirably other insurance cover should be taken out as well. A riding school must also comply with current employment and health and safety legislation. All these matters have been discussed in Chapter 5. Where residential facilities are provided for staff, students or clients, then the relevant food hygiene regulations must be observed.

The key to success is marketing which must ensure that the type of business suits the area. Any advertising is a waste of money if an establishment gets a bad reputation and customer satisfaction must be the objective. A key question is to ask oneself 'Did the client get value for money?' All too often it will be found that although the client gets value for money, the lesson did not give full satisfaction because the client expected something different. It is for this reason that it is important to listen to clients and also to educate them into having realistic expectations. Galloping through woodland with hair blowing in the breeze may not be a realistic expectation – particularly for a first lesson!

It is sensible for the riding school to seek approval from one of the horse/pony societies, each of which will provide full details of their approval scheme. Each scheme can be compared on its costs and merits and discussed with the proprietors of other riding schools. In some cases it is appropriate to seek approval under more than one scheme.

All the schemes require an inspection. The inspector's visit is advantageous in many ways, as he/she can bring an experienced view to bear on many aspects of the business as well as providing useful information about current trends and new developments. A society's annual conferences are good places to gain information.

The society's inspector is looking for a number of things. Once again, first impressions are important, but key elements in an initial or regrading inspection are shown in Table 9.3.

A riding school needs a good routine as discussed and illustrated in Chapter 7. The school should encompass the principles of student-centred learning set out in Chapter 3. It must be geared to give ample benefits to its clients, and they may have different expectations. This can be illustrated by some of the responses of customers of a particular riding school who were asked 'What do you expect from your riding lessons?' and, as can be seen from Table 9.4, the answers were many and varied.

Table 9.3 A typical checklist for an inspection of a riding establishment.

First impressions
- Well-signed off road.
- Direction sign to (a) car park, (b) reception.
- Tidy, well ordered yard.
- Fields well fenced, pasture in good order, troughs safe, shelter adequate.
- Staff friendly, who identify and greet strangers.

Lessons
- Appropriate standard, well organized, good instruction.
- Safe environment, safety tack check at start of lesson.
- Mounts: suitable, obedient, well schooled.
- Pupils: understand, learn progressively and enjoy.

Stable yard
- Horses and ponies: healthy, fit, good feet, if shod – shoes in good order.
- Stabling: good repair, safe.
- Isolation, sick treatment, fire provision, Incident Book.
- Good forage and bedding.
- Tack in good repair, clean, supple and suitable.

Teaching areas
- Good safe surface, level and not dusty.
- Safe area free from distraction or intrusion.
- 'Door drill' enforced.
- Suitable safe jumps.
- Safe gallery.

Accommodation
- Clean, dry, well lit and warm.
- Proper toilet facilities and plenty of hot water freely available.
- Rooms with adequate clothes storage and good beds.
- Kitchen hygienic with proper food storage provision.
- Clothes drying and laundry facility.

Riding school work

The provision of safe, suitable, willing and co-operative horses and ponies is essential to every riding school. If mounts are overworked they tend to become lame, thus putting pressure on others. Table 9.5 gives suggestions as to usage.

A good horse averaging 16 hours a week works 800 hours in a year. It will probably earn £100 a week, excluding the cost of the instructor.

Table 9.4 'What do you expect from your riding lessons?' The responses of customers at one riding school.

---

  (1) Learning to ride.
  (2) Enjoyment.
  (3) Fitness; helps strengthen the body.
  (4) Sense of achievement.
  (5) Physical and/or mental development.
  (6) Appeal to the competitive instinct.
  (7) Exams (qualification).
  (8) Improve ability.
  (9) Pleasure of teaching the horse.
(10) Outdoor activity.
(11) Country awareness.
(12) Develop 'feel'.
(13) Confidence.
(14) Joy of working with animals.
(15) Co-ordination.
(16) Fashionable.
(17) Prestige.
(18) Social gathering.
(19) Interest.
(20) For fun.
(21) For parents' ambitions.
(22) Aiming for a goal.
(23) Ambition.
(24) To sort out the horse's problem(s).
(25) Overcome fear.
(26) 'Because it's good for you.'
(27) Career
(28) Feeling of dominance (a) over the animal, (b) up on high.
(29) To go hunting.
(30) Snobbery.
(31) For greater safety.
(32) For a particular sport.
(33) Actors – need to ride.
(34) To exercise kids and/or pony.
(35) To understand the children.
(36) To help at RDA.
(37) 'Because I am a masochist.'

Riding school staff

Staff should not work long hours teaching; if they do, quality falls,

Table 9.5 Recommendations for horses and ponies for riding school work.

Type	Maximum total hours worked per week	Maximum hours per day	% spare horses	Accommodation pony	horse
Beginners	22	4.5	8%	Grass Barn	Grass Stall
Improvers	20	3.5	10%	Grass Stall	Grass Stall
Competent	18	3.0	12%	Grass Stall	Grass Box
Advanced	12	2.0	15%	Box	Box

sparkle is lost, individuality disappears and clients go elsewhere. Suggested maximum teaching hours might be 6 hours a day and 25 hours a week. This applies at all levels whether the teacher be an assistant, intermediate, instructor, trainer or fellow of the BHS.

Hacking is an important aspect of work in many riding schools, but much of the advice given below when discussing trekking is of equal application to hacking.

Trekking

The aim of trekking is to provide safe amusement on horseback to those who may not otherwise ride regularly or even at all. To be successful a trekking business must be well organized, well marketed, have good mounts and trek leaders and pleasant country with good access. Good organization should conform to the following plan:

(1) Riders should report to the reception area and be checked verbally and visually for their size, experience, expectations and suitability of dress.
(2) Cobs and ponies are allocated to the riders together with sound, safe and properly fitted tack.
(3) Riders' hats should be checked to ensure that they comply to BSI current standards, are in good condition, fit properly and are secured. Their footwear should be checked to ensure that it has a smooth sole and a good heel or that the saddle is kitted out with bucket stirrups

which the foot cannot slip through. Riders' trousers should be checked and leg protectors issued where necessary to prevent pinched calves. Jackets should be checked in view of possible weather conditions during the trek and their potential for startling horses by flapping.

(4) The riders should be installed on their mounts in a safe enclosed area and the correct match of mount and rider checked visually. They should then ride in a safe enclosed area to check their competence.

(5) The trek leader must be a competent rider aged at least 16 and preferably older. He/she must be able to supervise, give simple riding instructions and to administer both human and equine first aid. The leader should preferably have passed a test in riding and road safety and have a good knowledge and understanding of the country code. He/she should have good knowledge of local routes, conditions and people. (There is an examination and NVQ unit for trek leaders which provides a test of competence.)

The trek leader briefs the ride. The briefing should cover the following points:

- The trek leader is in charge.
- The planned route, pace and duration of the trek.
- Incident procedure. This should include how to cope with accidents and possible emergencies.
- The other staff going on the trek.

(6) The trek then takes place to an agreed and logged plan, and its design and execution should give pleasure to the least able. Whatever the weather, the ride should be a happy affair enjoyed by all participants. The ride must never over-stretch the riders' competence. The number of escorts should be:

- One for each six clients at faster pace – cantering and with some jumps.
- One for each seven clients at medium pace – trotting and some cantering.
- One for each eight clients at slow pace – walking and some trots.

The total number of clients in a ride should not exceed 20. Front and rear riders should be responsible. The trek leader or escorts should carry first aid gear and small change for the telephone. A small mobile telephone may be useful.

(7) When the riders return, the horses and tack should be put away and any loaned or hired clothing retrieved.

(8) The log book should be completed and any incidents noted. Major incidents must be fully recorded in the Incident Book.

Farmers who are considering entering the trekking business may find that grants are available to them: ADAS can advise. The major problem in running a trekking centre is in the seasonal nature of the activity. Staff may be engaged on a seasonal basis, but reliable mounts need to be retained. Large numbers of horses have to be kept cheaply out of season, which requires a farm or grazing rights. Alternatively, the horses can be sent away to a farm which will take a block booking of six months at cheap rates. Because of this it follows that native stock or native cross mounts are essential so that they are economical to keep and will overwinter without problems in fairly tough conditions.

Rights of way

Any stables offering hacking or trekking facilities need access to good riding and this entails rights of way since there is no right to ride over someone else's land without permission. The local highway authority is responsible for all rights of way and these are shown on Ordnance Survey Pathfinder Maps (4 cm to 1 km or 2.5 in to 1 mile). A definitive map of all rights of way is maintained at the offices of the county council. A bridleway is a highway over which the public have a right of way on foot and on horseback or leading a horse. They are usually signed with blue arrows while byways open to all traffic are waymarked red. Horses are not allowed on to footpaths which are waymarked yellow unless the landowner consents. Gates on bridleways should be at least 1.53 m (5 ft) wide and this can be enforced by the highway authority. A farmer can plough up a bridleway which crosses a field but not one on a headland. Even if the ground is ploughed and sown, the right of way still exists. Any interference with a right of way (or attempted intimidation of its users) should be reported to the authority, as should any misleading notice. Unfortunately, not all highway authorities are as diligent as they might be in maintaining bridleways or in enforcing the rights of the public. Riders may take a short cut round an illegal obstruction on a right of way or remove it sufficiently to clear a path. .

In the interests of riding generally, the best plan is to ride bridleways and help to clear them while earning the goodwill of landowners. Riders should join their local British Horse Society Bridleways group. By their responsible attitude and consideration for others, horse riders should be welcome wherever there is suitable riding.

Accommodation

Accommodation for clients is an important enterprise, especially associated with trekking centres, but it is also linked with riding schools and other equine businesses. Needless to say, the statutory regulations relating to fire precautions and hygiene must be complied with. If the establishment is a member of an association, there will be an association code of conduct to be adhered to.

The establishment must set its own style in terms of luxury or simplicity, and what is offered must be made plain in any literature sent out. Courtesy of service and a desire to provide clients with an enjoyable stay should be universal. Cleanliness and hygiene should be of exemplary standards, but the degree of decoration and the sophistication of the decor should follow the chosen style. Amenities, facilities and services provided should all be fairly and accurately described in any leaflets. The price must be clearly shown and there should be no hidden extras so that clients receive the bill they anticipated and not an inflated one. If the main accommodation is full and alternative arrangements such as housing in an annexe are available, the client should be advised and asked for agreement in advance. The range of accommodation arrangements varies from double-bunk dormitories with self-catering (youth hostel style) to luxurious apartments with fine menus. In general, providing beds is more profitable than providing food. A bed and breakfast with packed lunch or a snack bar may be complemented by evening meals at the local public house.

Serious consideration should be given to the provision of a caravan and camping ground. It will earn money in its own right and will bring in extra clients or allow clients to stay on site at reasonable cost. Expansion to provide site caravans for holidaymakers and the provision of permanent toilets and washing blocks is a possibility in the right area, assuming the hurdle of planning permission can be overcome. Tourist-related expansion may be eligible for Tourist Board grants.

Studs

British studs offer an immense variety of levels and styles. There are sumptuous studs on large private estates – one stud has 12 miles of private roads. Others operate as a quiet sideline to the main equestrian business. Britain bred the thoroughbred which is the racehorse of the world and our thoroughbred breeding is still brilliant, sophisticated and a source of great national pride. Britain's native ponies are another part of our heritage and are cared for by dedicated breeders and the breed societies, although being part of Europe may present problems for some of these. Our breeding of Arabs (both as show horses and race horses) shows a considerable understanding and appreciation of world bloodlines. Britain's native heavy horses – the Shire, the Clydesdale and the Suffolk – are exported and greatly admired for their quality. The great national sport of hunting gives us the opportunity to performance test horses in a unique way, but it is in the breeding of performance horses that Britain has lost ground. Past policy has been to distribute race horse stallions around the country and to judge the progeny as 'hunters' in the show ring. British competitors often need to buy performance horses in other European countries which have followed the sensible pattern used in racing, i.e. the combination of performance testing with progeny testing. A stud wishing to achieve commercial success in a highly competitive market should consider these aspects of the subject.

Performance testing is to test the animal's performance against strictly defined criteria and see how well it performs. The success of the method depends on how well the criteria are set, how scrupulously the tests are operated, how well the records are kept, and how carefully the information is used to breed future generations. If the test set is to win in the show ring, then it is a matter of subjective individual judgement as opinions may vary and tastes may change. A more objective test is likely to ensure that performance is likely to improve over the years. Progeny testing is to test the performance of the offspring and to credit the parent accordingly so achieving a higher price. Racing has long used this approach and has combined both performance and progeny testing in attempting to breed the stars of the future. Similarly, European breed societies have worked out and followed such a system which relies on guaranteed identification of every horse and comprehensive central records. Individual judgement still has a part to play in that each horse is still required to be a fine physical specimen with excellent conformation and a suitable temperament.

Breeding horses is expensive. Many of the costs – land, feed, labour and overheads – will be the same for a good specimen as for a mediocre one. The costs involved are generally such as to make it difficult to show a profit on the average horse or pony. Such animals are bred for love or as a sideline where the full cost can be hidden. A prosperous stud must put the accent on *excellence* and *success*. Breeding policy is the first critical aspect of stud management. To market a stallion at stud, for example, it must be shown that he comes from good lines of proven performers on both sides and also that he is a fine specimen and a good performer in his own right. The stallion must also produce stock which are good performers.

Marketing is also important to stud management. It is not enough to have the best stallion; the clients have got to be persuaded to send their mares to the stallion. Potential clients must read sufficient in the advertisements to make them send for the stallion's stud card. Just as in other areas, any literature must be well-produced and persuade clients to visit the stud. They will have come partly to see the stallion, but will also hope to see some of his progeny – if not in the flesh, then certainly in photographs. Customers also need to be impressed by the hygiene, good stockmanship and attention to detail.

The stud's marketing policy is also concerned with selling the progeny at a good price. Continental sales again provide superb examples of how all breeders can benefit through a well thought out marketing campaign which includes prestige sales based on selection for performance.

Where a stud chooses to breed thoroughbreds, the entire pattern is well-established. Likewise, if the stud is to breed pure-breds for the show ring, each breed will have its own principal shows and sales. The stud may have to gain success in the show ring to gain credibility.

In the breeding of performance horses, many British light draught breeds have been allowed to become extinct in recent years. Examples are the Norfolk Roadster – perfect for long distance riding; the Yorkshire Coach Horse and the Devon Pack Horse. Such bloodlines have been carefully preserved in Continental Europe and have been blended with thoroughbred inputs for quality. At present, Britain is importing warm bloods. Soon, however, this imported blood together with our Cleveland, Irish Draught and Hunter blood will provide all the material needed for British high performance horses to be as much sought after as the German, Dutch and Danish performance horses are.

Further information is set out in John Rose and Sarah Pilliner's book: *Breeding the Competition Horse* Second Edition (Blackwell Science).

Tack shop

A tack shop is one of the most common enterprises to be run with a riding school. A do-it-yourself livery yard can also take advantage of the clients on site and extend their product range to include the hay, concentrates and bedding which the clients need to purchase. The tack shop can have restricted hours and at a riding school can be operated by the school's receptionist.

The major difficulty with a tack shop is that the retail business requires expertise which may be lacking among the horse staff. If the shop is sufficiently large to employ a specialist, he/she will understand about stock control and the other necessary skills of retailing. Someone lacking that experience may find that they cannot attract customers because the shop has insufficient stock to meet the customers' needs or that they cannot afford to carry a large amount of stock.

On average, each stock item will sit on the shelf for four to five months, and although some items will move more quickly, others will be slower. The stock must be of the style and range to suit the majority of potential customers. Stock need not necessarily be an equestrian item; giftware may be appropriate for a trekking centre, for example. In order to stock the shop, it is necessary to find a good wholesaler and this can be done through the British Equestrian Trade Association.

Usually the goods can be sold at any price the retailer chooses; very few items have a recommended retail price. In the saddlery trade, a mark-up of up to 100 per cent is common. This provides a good living for the larger establishments but is necessary for survival in the smaller ones. VAT is added on top of the mark-up. Regular customers and riding club members may think that they are entitled to a discount. However, discounts are like bonus payments – they can rebound and soon everyone thinks that they are entitled to a percentage off.

Those staffing the shop must understand the technical side of the use of any products which they sell. They must also have the personality which makes a customer feel happy to have visited the shop. However, not all visitors will be welcome and the retail trade suffers hugely from theft (euphemistically called 'shoplifting') and so central stands which hide customers with shopping bags or loose-fitting jackets should be avoided. Experienced staff – aided by corner mirrors – should keep an eye on stock. Strong grilles and locks together with an intruder detection system may be essential. A proper till, a safe and a routine for transferring money to the bank regularly are all part of the business of retail selling. The shop should be run as a separate business and planning permission may well be necessary. However, in the right area and with the right stock and marketing, a shop can suitably complement another horse business.

10 Special events

Open days

All equestrian businesses need to organize special events from time to
time, and 'open days' are one of the most popular. They can be wildly
successful. A racing yard in the Cotswolds has a regular attendance of
about 4,000 on its annual open day. A Berkshire stud has to insist on
advance bookings and run several performances because its open day is
so popular. At open days like this, members of the public are willing to
pay to attend, largely because of the quality of the entertainment and
relaxation provided and the charisma of the owner/presenters. Another
stud, attracting similar numbers to its open day, combines it with a village
open day and has again established a spot in the local annual calendar of
events. It takes time to build up a reputation of this sort, but much
depends on the quality of the first open day which is organized.

Unless the owner of the business is a well-known equestrian personality, then a 'star' may have to be imported. This might be a well-known
person or a famous horse. The open day must have a purpose, which is
normally publicity for the business. Advertising the open day is also a
good promotion for the business. The day's programme or brochure can
carry advertisements, and these may be solicited from those who trade
with the business, including the bank, the solicitors, the estate agents
involved when it was purchased, as well as the vet, the farrier and feed
merchant and others who have become involved with it. Local traders in
the area may be persuaded to place advertisements, as may specialist
shops such as local saddlers, horsebox manufacturers and so on.
Generally, the public will be willing to pay an admission charge, but there
will be many people who ought to be sent complimentary tickets. Even if
they do not actually attend on the day, the business will have gained much
goodwill merely for the price of printing and posting the invitations.

A small business just launching into the marketplace may find it
difficult to put on a worthwhile show, but with imagination the

programme can be expanded. The trade stands which are found at horse events may be persuaded to set up in a concourse or shopping area. A local star dressage rider might provide elegance with a dressage to music display, and this might contrast well with something like a costumed quadrille team riding to lively western or folk music. A side-saddle rider might explain the intricacies of her art and give a demonstration. Lungeing and long-reining accompanied by a well-informed commentary can be interesting and educational. The nature of the business must be the central theme, and a well-illustrated printed programme can be used not only for reference during the event but for subsequent reference and a reminder of the business.

An open day involves a great deal of hard work. It requires much mowing, trimming, painting and polishing. Flower tubs and hanging baskets may need to be hired to supplement those on the premises. While fine weather is to be hoped for, wet weather must be provided for. Open days are only put on by the brave but, if done well, they can contribute to the success of a business by enhancing its reputation.

Shows

Shows of various sorts invariably attract interest, but before organizing one, various factors need to be considered, not least the administration involved. It is easy to be talked into organizing a show, but it is best not to embark on the project without considerable research and thought.

The first point is to consider why the show is needed. Who wants the show? Is it being put on for competitors, or the organizers, or the spectators, or a mix of the three? Who will gain from the show? Is it being run for a cause or is it designed to increase the profitability of the business? The next point for consideration is what sort of show is to be organized and how the classes are to be mixed. Which organizations the show should seek affiliation with is also an important question, as is the size of the show itself. How the show is to be organized is the next point for decision. A show can be run by one person, a committee or even by a professional organizer; the latter will want a fee.

The choice of venue must then be considered. This may be obvious as it may be dictated by the business premises. However, there may be choices to be made, especially if a joint venture with others is a possibility. The choice of venue can be dictated by facilities available or influenced by the necessary amenities and the cost of hiring items. Finally, the timing of the show must be decided. In many disciplines, national programmes have to be taken into account. Local links must be forged because every area has its own local programme of annual events. 'Local' in this context may spread over more than one county.

Once the show is over, the financial and non-financial aspects of the venture must be carefully considered. At the planning stage, a budget will have been prepared, and likely headings for the income and expenditure account are:

Income	Expenditure
Entry fees.	Affiliation fees. Levies.
Entrance fees/parking.	Advertising (including signs).
Sale of programmes.	Insurance. Rosettes. Score sheets.
Trade stands.	Police. AA.
Sponsorship.	Printing and stationery.
Advertising.	Hire and preparation of ground.
Refreshments.	Judges' and first aiders' expenses.
Raffle tickets.	Postage and telephone.
	Refunds and prize money.
	Refreshments and meals for officials.
	Arena party.
	Course construction and repair.
	Making good and cleaning the show ground.
	Hire of jumps, judges, boxes, timing, toilets, ropes and posts, marquees, arenas, public address, score boards, etc.
	Doctor, vet, farrier.

The headings are not comprehensive – and much the same balance sheet applies to any special event. Intangible benefits for the organizing establishment flow from the publicity and potential extra business, which must be offset against notional or actual income lost because of the time spent on administration and the disruptive effect of the event. Many shows only break even in financial terms.

Reasons for repeating the show might be:

- It was good publicity and a prestigious event.
- It was good public relations.
- It was an achievement.
- It was enjoyable.
- It entertained clients and others.
- It made money.

In contrast, reasons for not repeating the experiment include:

- It disrupted the existing business.
- It caused serious damage to the ground and excessive wear and tear.
- It was not appreciated.
- It lost money.
- Neighbours complained.

Many of these are personal factors and the ultimate decision is not necessarily logical. Shows certainly have a place as special events and can produce results for the business, even if they are not represented in an immediate cash return.

Cross-country

Organizing a cross-country event is another possibility, provided one has the ground, as well as the administrative ability and other skills involved. It is not only the design of the course itself which is important; many other matters must be considered as part of the overall plan:

- Car parking.
- Lorry park – on downhill slope with bottom exit.
- Dressage areas – well away from the cross-country course.
- Show jumping arena and practice area.
- Secretary – convenient to the lorry park.
- Commentator.
- Scorers – convenient to the score board.
- Toilets.
- Refreshments.
- First aid – ambulance access to all fences.

The cross-country course itself is critical to success and should be designed with its most ambitious feature in mind. The course is usually a permanent feature. The most obvious piece of ground for a cross-country course may have intrusive features or have to accommodate other facilities as well. The applicable rules must be checked for the distance and number of fences and their height and type. Other uses for the fences, such as training, must be considered and if space permits it is best to have both a cross-country course and a training ground.

Three points are paramount in course design:

(1) Tracks of the required distance on the best-drained available land and with good viewing for the commentator and spectators.

(2) Selected fence sites on the track. Groups of fences add to spectator interest, as do areas where the horses can be seen outward and homeward. Making the track deviate to take in a special feature often spoils the flow of the course.
(3) Create a course which looks good and rides well. Obstacles should be designed to offer a good selection of a few uprights, plenty of spreads, banks, ditches and combinations. Fences can be related to turns and other natural features.

Fence-designing allows for some individuality, but the standard constructional features of all cross-country fences are based on experience. The novice course-builder should not be too innovative. A good fence has important hallmarks:

- It looks right and suits the spot. Good use is made of natural and local materials. The fence is well related to natural features and to the course as a whole.
- The fence is bold, simple and clear. Big timber helps create the bold look, as does good width. Twenty feet wide looks more than twice as good as ten! Big timber also gives strength; this is important because the course must be the same for the last horse as it is for the first one. There should be no hold-ups or calls for a fence repair party. Telegraph poles and railway sleepers lend themselves to fence construction.
- The fence encourages young horses to jump freely and in good style. It may require both horse and rider to use their intelligence but will never be 'trappy'.
- The fence will be safe: a horse stopping, slipping or sliding into or onto the jump can always be removed quickly by cutting securing ropes with an axe. Pen fences and wide ditches should have walk-out areas for horses which stop or fall into them.
- The fence will test both horse and rider to a defined and specified standard and must be designed for that purpose. Scaled-down international fences do not necessarily make good novice fences.
- The fence will be sited on well-drained ground which will not get too deep. Approach and landing must both be good. Walking round the course in summertime may well prove misleading if the fence is to be jumped in the spring after a wet winter.
- The fence will be fair to all. A related fence involving a tight turn will favour the pony type. A combination fence with a long stride favours the bigger horses. The course may contain a collection of different tests, but the overall balance should not favour any type.
- Attention to detail is essential. For example, it is insufficient merely to

cut off a post to the correct height; the cut edge must be chamfered so that it is smooth and safe. Permanent timber fences should be creosoted yearly so that they look dark, smart and imposing. The fences can be dressed with carefully positioned fir trees: this makes a great deal of difference to the course.

- Where funds are limited, a short and simple course built to a high standard is better than a more complicated course in which standards are low.

A training ground is also needed (Figs 10.1 and 10.2); this does not require much space or big fences, but its design is also important. The aim

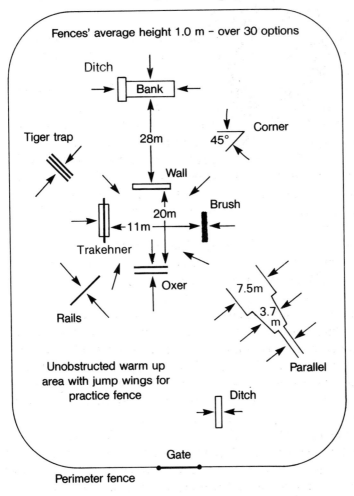

Fig. 10.1 Cross-country training complex.

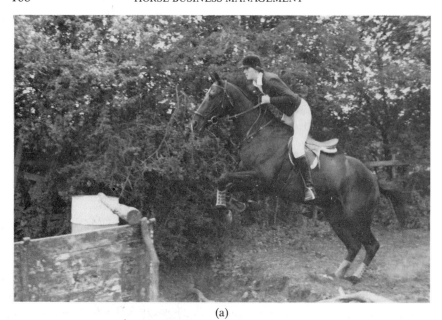

(a)

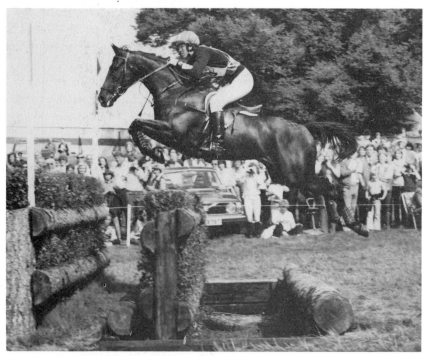

(b)

Fig. 10.2 (a) Simple ditches and rails in the training field prepare the young horse; (b) the same horse with the same rider when they reach international standard.

is to improve the confidence and performance of both horse and rider. It can be used to practise approaches at different length of strides and different angles. It can be so ridden that riders land and turn sharply between cones or come between cones and turn sharply leaving only a short approach to the fence. Cross-country training fences will get much use and so need hard-wearing take-offs and landings. The training ground will need refurbishment more often than the cross-country course itself.

Show jumping

Show jumping continues to be popular and it has an active and vigilant organizing body in the British Show Jumping Association (BSJA). It is not surprising, therefore, that most commercial enterprises with indoor arenas of sufficient size are tempted to put on a jumping show in the winter, and throughout the summer there are local jumping shows of every type and level. There are over 2,000 shows in Britain between March and October plus indoor jumping throughout the winter.

In organizing a jumping show, an important consideration is that horseboxes and trailers take up a lot of space. They need wide entrances and exits with safe vision. Another important point is that while there is only one horse in the main jumping ring at any one time, there may be ten or more in the practice area. Ample space and good going are therefore important. Poor facilities at indoor shows often deter potential competitors.

A good jumping show requires a good organizing team able to work together. They are the judge, the judge's writer, the timekeeper, the announcer, the collecting ring steward, the course builder and the arena party. An experienced judge can train his/her team in the box and a good course builder can train both the arena party and advise the steward. The manager of the business must ensure that the show keeps up to standard and may be asked to advise on various points, but the judge is responsible for all happenings in the ring and his/her authority must be maintained.

The judge's box must not become a social area and those wishing to speak to the judge should only do so between classes or rounds. Judging involves much concentration and distracted judges make mistakes and the show loses credibility.

The announcer sets the tone of the show. He/she welcomes everyone at the outset, announces the classes and results, and mentions the sponsors as appropriate. At the end of the day the announcer thanks all those involved. Announcers should not caution or admonish competitors over the public address system nor should they make sarcastic or facetious remarks.

Course building

The course builder's aim is to build an attractive course which will keep the spectators' and competitors' attention. Well-built courses produce exciting contests. Each horse should enjoy its round and learn from the experience. The riders should gain a sense of achievement in completing the course, and eliminations should be avoided as much as possible.

So that the course builder can achieve success, certain information is needed:

- the schedule of classes;
- anticipated number of starters in each class;
- target timetable;
- standard of competitors and mounts;
- ideal number of clear rounds in each class;
- non-jumping events which will take place in the ring.

The course builder also needs details of the ring or arena itself and ideally should visit the area. Critical features are its size, location of the judge's box and of the entrance and exit. The course builder must also have details of the show jumps available, practice fences and available decoration. If appropriate, there must be provision for hard ground. The time for building the course must be agreed.

Length of the track and the site of the start and finish of the course are critical factors to smooth operation. Start and early fences should head towards 'home' (the collecting ring) so as to get the horses off to a fluent start. The layout of the course should allow a second horse to enter the arena before the previous one has finished. The finish should not gallop horses straight out of the exit, but be so arranged that when a horse has finished the course and pulled up it is near to the exit.

The course must have a good track; it must flow. The actual design and relationship of fences requires experience. The greatest care must be taken with distances. Good going, downhill gradients and lines towards 'home' require slightly longer distances. Poor going, uphill gradients, soon after corners and courses indoors may require slightly shorter distances. The BSJA publishes detailed information about the best distances. Table 10.1 is a useful guide.

Table 10.1 A guide to distances.

	ft	m
Two non-jumping strides		
Experienced horses	34.5	10.5
Low jumps and novice horses	33.0	10.1
Experienced ponies 14.2 hh	33.0	10.1
Experienced ponies 13.2 hh	32.5	9.9
Experienced ponies 12.2 hh	32.0	9.7
One non-jumping stride		
Experienced horses	23.0–24.5	7.0–7.5
Low jumps and novice horses	21.5–23.0	6.5–7.0
Experienced ponies 14.2 hh	22.5–23.0	6.8–7.0
Experienced ponies 13.2 hh	22.0–22.5	6.7–6.8
Experienced ponies 12.2 hh	21.5–22.0	6.5–6.7
(the shorter distance is for a spread fence going out)		
Three non-jumping horse strides	47.0	14.3
Four non-jumping horse strides	58.0	17.7
Five non-jumping horse strides	69.0	21.0
(reduce by at least a foot for indoors)		

Appendix 1: Guidance on promoting safe working conditions

Based on notes prepared by the Health and Safety Executive.

PART A – GENERAL ADVICE FOR ALL HORSE ESTABLISHMENTS

A1   Introduction

The purpose of this note is to give practical guidance on promoting safe working conditions at horse establishments and to assist those persons concerned to fulfil their statutory duties under the Health and Safety at Work etc. Act 1974.

Most accidents at horse establishments arise from riding and handling horses. Horses are unpredictable but implementing good systems of work minimizes the risk.

A2   Legislation

A2.1   Employers, employees and the self-employed have far reaching duties under the Health and Safety at Work etc. Act 1974. Employers must do everything reasonably practicable to ensure the health, safety and welfare of their employees.

A2.2   In addition, employers and the self-employed must do everything reasonably practicable to ensure their own safety and that of other people who are not their employees but who may be affected by the work activity.

Close communication should be maintained with contractors where their normal operations could heighten the risk of accidents in the work place. Particularly, contractors should be made aware of the easily-frightened nature of horses.

A2.3   Duties are placed on persons having control, to any extent, of non-domestic premises, used by people who are not their employees. These duties apply when people enter to work there or where machinery or substances are provided for their use.

A2.4   Those who manage and operate horse establishments therefore have a duty not only to their own and other people's employees working at these premises but also to visitors there and to members of the public outside whose health and safety may be affected.

It should be noted that children or inexperienced people may inadvertently place themselves in danger where an experienced person would recognize the risks.

A2.5   Employees must take reasonable care to avoid injury to themselves and to others by their work activities and must co-operate with employers and others in fufiling statutory requirements.

Failure to comply with safety regulations can lead to grounds for dismissal. Employees also have a duty to report shortcomings in arrangements for safety.

A2.6   Although horse establishments conduct a specialized activity, many of the essential safety requirements are not unlike those necessary at other farm livestock rearing premises. Relevant health and safety standards already exist in the form of agricultural legislation and other guidance, applicable to, for example, the construction and maintenance of buildings, storage and use of veterinary products and disinfectants, installation and maintenance of electrical fixtures and fittings, storage and use of LPG (liquefied petroleum gas), welfare facilities, and provision and maintenance of safe plant and equipment. Regulations and standards can be used as a guide to enable persons to fulfil obligations under the General Duties sections of the Health and Safety at Work etc. Act 1974. Emphasis should be placed on safe systems of work.

A3   Management of health and safety

Health and safety is not only required by law, it also makes economic sense. No business can easily afford to have a key employee unavailable for work. To be successful the adoption of safe working practices has to be managed. Consultation with employees and close observation of normal work practices enable a detailed risk assessment to be completed for every aspect of workplace activity.

Risk assessment should not be a discrete undertaking, it needs to be a continuous process to account for changes in activity and circumstances. A thorough risk assessment develops into a policy statement.

A3.1   Policy statements.

A3.2 Where five or more people are employed, the Act places a duty on an employer to prepare and as often as may be appropriate revise a written statement of his general policy with respect to the health and safety at work of his employees, and for the organization and arrangements for the time being in force for carrying out that policy, and to bring the statement and any revision of it to the notice of all of his employees. An employer should include part-time, casual and self-employed workers as part of the five or more employees.

A3.3 Written safety policy statements may be considered as being in three parts:
(a) the statement of the employer's general policy with regard to the health and safety of his employees;
(b) the organization for carrying out the policy; and
(c) the arrangements for carrying out the policy.

A3.4 The statement should cover the intent to comply with current statutory provisions and should lay particular emphasis on safe work routines. It should stress the importance of co-operation from the workforce and of good communications at all levels in the business. The statement should be signed by the employer or a partner or senior director.

A3.5 Where necessary the statement should clearly define the responsibilities of named senior and junior members of staff with regard to health and safety generally, and to emergency situations. Those named must have adequate information and authority to perform their responsibilities.

A3.6 It is important that any likely hazards and the extent of health and safety matters under the employer's control are identified. Hazards can be listed together with the rules and precautions for avoiding them and arrangements for dealing with injury, fire and other emergencies should be made clear. The arrangements for providing instruction, training and supervision should also be identified.

A3.7 The general policy must be monitored and kept under review and the statement amended where necessary. The original statement and any subsequent revision must be brought to the notice of all employees. Newly recruited employees should not be overlooked.

A3.8 Each employer must write his policy statement according to his own needs. It must be emphasized that the written word does not prevent accidents and it is the thorough implementation of an effective policy that can play an important part in accident prevention.

A3.9 The priced Health and Safety Executive booklet *Writing Your Health and Safety Policy Statement* is available from HMSO (ISBN 0 11885510 7). It gives guidance on the preparation of a statement, laying out the important points using page by page examples.

A4   Washing and sanitary facilities

A4.1   Suitable and sufficient washing and sanitary facilities should be available to all employees. (Further guidance is given at Annex 2.)

A4.2   Where male and female workers are employed, one sanitary convenience is adequate providing the total number of employees does not exceed five. Where the workforce exceeds five, facilities should be provided in relation to the numbers of workers employed as follows:

Number of workers	Number of water closets	Number of washing stations
1–5	1	1
6–25	2	2
26–50	3	3
51–75	4	4
76–100	5	5

A4.3   Sanitary facilities must be under cover, partitioned off for privacy, have adequate lighting and have proper doors and fastenings. They must not communicate directly with a room or place in which people are working. The interior of a room housing a sanitary convenience must not be visible – even with the door open – by members of the opposite sex, and urinals must not be visible from any place where people work or pass. Sanitary facilities must be maintained, kept clean and have an adequate supply of paper. Where female facilities are provided, suitable means for the disposal of sanitary dressings should be available.

A4.4   Wherever it is reasonably practicable to do so, water closets (WCs) or urinals should be provided. Where this is not practicable, a chemical or dry packaging toilet may be used.

A4.5   Washbasins must include clean running hot (or warm) and cold water, soap (liquid, powder or solid), drying facilities (continuous linen towels, disposable paper towels, automatic hot air dryers, etc.). The facilities must be conveniently accessible to the workforce and must be kept in a clean and orderly condition.

A4.6   Rest rooms are particularly important to those working outside for long periods. They should be large enough to accommodate the number of employees likely to be using them at any one time. Arrangements should be made to allow separate areas for smokers and non-smokers.

A5   First-aid and occupational health

A5.1   Minimum standards for the provision of first-aid are contained in the Health and Safety (First-Aid) Regulations 1981. The priced booklet *First-Aid at Work* HS(R) 11 obtainable from HMSO gives guidance in this respect.

A5.2   It is recommended that all establishments should have at least one person available who has received training in occupational first-aid and is a certified first-aider. First-aid stations should be clearly identified, and appropriate first-aid materials must be maintained.

A5.3   Any staff or other persons who ride or come into contact with horses on the premises should be encouraged to seek immunization against tetanus.

A5.4   To reduce the risk of contracting Weil's disease (leptospirosis), persons required to work in areas which have been contaminated by rodents should be provided with suitable protective clothing and advised on standards of personal hygiene. An effective rodent control programme should also be carried out whenever the need arises.

A5.5   Taking care in the purchase, preparation and storage of feedstuffs or bedding minimizes the formation of harmful organisms which may be the cause of farmer's lung or other respiratory ailments. Persons required to work in dusty conditions, or to handle mouldy hay or straw, should be provided with suitable respiratory protection which is cheaply available from an agricultural merchant.

A5.6   The Reporting of Injuries, Diseases and Dangerous Occurrences Regulations 1985 (RIDDOR) require employers to report certain types of injury, disease or accidents. Reports must be made to the local environmental health department. The regulations are complex and further detail can be found in the Health and Safety Executive booklet HS(R)23. However, briefly they are as follows:

> If there is an accident at work which results in death or a member of staff being off work for more than three days, or major bones are broken (not fingers or toes), or an eye is damaged, or a part of the body is amputated, or there is unconsciousness or injury due to an electric shock or lack of oxygen or absorption of a substance (by eating it, drinking it, breathing it or having it on the skin), or if there is acute illness from bacteria or fungi or other infected material, or if the person has to go to hospital for more than 24 hours, then the matter must be reported to the local environmental health department at once.

Ask Directory Enquiries or the local district council office for the telephone number. If in doubt, phone and ask advice. They will send forms for completion. It is an offence not to report such an accident.

Also under the same regulations certain diseases must be reported; these include asthma caused by working in dusty conditions, farmer's lung and leptospirosis (Weil's disease).

A6   Machinery, equipment and premises

A6.1   All machinery and equipment should be installed, used and maintained in such a way that it does not present a hazard and that its safe operation cannot be interfered with.

A6.2   Many horse establishments have a wide range of agricultural machinery. Care should be taken to ensure that such machines are guarded to an appropriate standard and are only used by persons who have received the necessary training and instruction in their correct use. Visitors or members of the general public are not to be exposed to risk when machinery is in operation.

A6.3   Those buildings, structures and areas to which it is necessary for employees and visitors to have access should be so designed and maintained that they offer no danger to a person in or in the vicinity of them. Access to upper or lower areas should be by permanent stairways or ladders with suitable hand-rails and hand-holds. Where access is needed only occasionally, a portable, safely placed or secured ladder may be used. Floor surfaces should be anti-slip and free draining with open edges guarded or fenced where a person is liable to fall more than 1.5 m.

A7   Provision of specialist equipment

Such equipment may include lifting tackle, 'carousels' for horse exercise and swimming pools. Lifting tackle, together with any ropes and slings, should be adequate for the purpose, properly maintained and regularly examined by a competent person. In all cases, manufacturers' instructions are to be observed. Carousels which are driven by electric motors need to be adequately earthed and suitably protected. Where a horse swimming pool is used, in addition to suitably fenced walkways around the edge of the pool, there should be adequate means of access and egress and appropriate rescue equipment. Unauthorized persons should not have access to the pool area.

A8   Manual handling

The work of attending horses may involve lifting or moving relatively heavy weights or awkward loads and training in lifting and carrying techniques is essential. If the load is too heavy for one person to lift, assistance must be sought. Lifting and moving aids should be used wherever possible, and such aids should be kept in good condition and well maintained. Where supervised young persons

- *Assess the situation:*
  Dress – boots, gloves, etc.
  Equipment – pitch fork, bale hook, pulley, trolley, jack, lever, etc.
  Assistance – machine, team, mate, etc.
  Reconnoitre – safe object, safe route, safe landing zone, safe weight.

- *Stance:*
  Feet apart – balanced; one foot forward.
  As close as possible to the object.
  Back straight, chin in.
  Legs bent.

- *Grip (lifting from floor):*
  Hand close and under weight or object clutched close to body.

- *Vision:*
  Do not block your view.

- *Lift:*
  Up and forwards – use leg muscles (calves, thighs, buttocks) but *not* back muscles.
  Do *not* twist or bend your spine.
  Keep weight close to body.

- *Carry:*
  Do not hurry, easy breathing, short steps.

- *Deposit:*
  Reverse of lift.

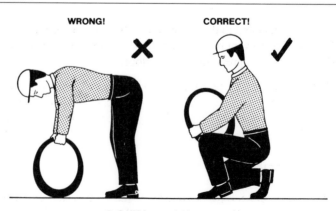

Safe lifting technique.

are allowed to assist, great care needs to be taken to ensure that they are not exposed to risks.

An assessment of lifting and carrying operations is particularly important where loads are flexible (e.g. feed sacks), bulky or where the working environment poses hazards in itself. Stacking bales of hay and straw poses particular risk. The load is bulky, strings may be insecure, the bales already in place offer a poor footing and visibility may be impaired.

The diagram and checklist opposite will help to avoid injury during lifting operations.

A9 Stabling

A9.1 Consideration needs to be given to the construction and dimensions of stables not only for the safety of personnel but also for the well-being of the horse. Stabling should be of adequate size, well ventilated, with sufficient head room provided and care taken to ensure that this is maintained if a deep litter type of bedding system is adopted.

A9.2 Ideally doors should be in two halves, outward opening, not less than 1.35 m (4 ft 6 in) wide with galvanized mouldings and kicking boards. Both doors should be fitted with anti-slide bolts with a kick latch at the base of the lower door. Walls should be clear of nails or other obstructions which may cause injury to either horse or person. It is recommended that areas under feed and drinking troughs are infilled. A safe means of securing the horse in the stable should be provided. Where windows are fitted with glass, protection bars should be fitted to prevent breakage.

A9.3 Stable floors should be soundly constructed, free from obstruction and provide an adequate foot-hold for both horse and handler. If concrete is to be laid, herring-bone or similar grooving should be incorporated for both anti-slip and drainage purposes.

A9.4 It is recommended that the top half of the opening door to a stallion box is suitably fenced to prevent risk of injury to passers-by. This applies to any horse which shows signs of aggression over the door.

A9.5 A clear area with adequate foot-hold should be provided outside the stable, free from any obstruction or distraction which could upset the horse, with all entry and exit points suitably gated to prevent loose horses escaping.

A10 Food preparation areas

A10.1 Hot water boilers are often used in the preparation of rations. These should be maintained and operated safely and in accordance with manufacturers' instructions, with the necessary equipment and protective clothing provided for staff to avoid the risk of injury.

A11 Hostels

Establishments providing hostel accommodation for employees should consult the local Fire Authority with regard to the provision of a current fire certificate. Depending on the type and situation of hostel accommodation, inspection by the local authority may also be required.

A12 Fire

A12.1 Most premises are particularly prone to fire hazards. Buildings are often constructed largely of wood, with hay and straw liberally used, and therefore smoking should be prohibited. Suitable fire precautions are a condition of the licence required under the Riding Establishments Act. The advice of the local Fire Prevention Officer should be followed in all matters of fire prevention and the provision of suitable fire fighting aids which should be subject to regular inspection by a competent person.

A12.2 Employers should ascertain if the Fire Precautions Act 1971 applies to their situation, e.g. where hostel accommodation is provided. Such premises should be in possession of a current Fire Certificate (hostels may also be subject to inspection by the local authority).

A12.3 Most horses are terrified by fire and can be difficult to lead out of a stable. It is therefore suggested that head collars are kept outside stables to facilitate quick removal in the event of fire. Additionally, a coat, blanket or similar article placed over the horse's head, covering the eyes but not the nostrils, will help when leading a horse near fire.

A12.4 A suitable secure paddock, known to all members of staff, should be kept free of unnecessary obstructions, securely gated and available for containing all horses during an emergency.

A12.5 Procedures in the event of fire should be clearly defined, brought to the attention of staff and adequately displayed for the benefit of both staff and visitors. Fire notices should comply with the Riding Establishments Acts 1964 and 1970. Fire drills and demonstrations of the use of fire fighting equipment are invaluable.

A13 Electricity

A13.1 Maintenance of all electrical equipment and new installations should be in accordance with the current IEE Wiring Regulations. Inspection/Certification of the installation by a competent person should be at regular intervals and not less than once every three years.

A13.2   Suitable and properly maintained residual current circuit breakers should be installed, particularly in areas where pressure washers or steam equipment are used. All electrical switches, sockets and wiring both within and outside stables should be located so that contact by horses is avoided. Where practicable, electrically operated hand tools, e.g. clippers, should be at a reduced voltage, 110 CTE and provided with non-detachable flexible cable incorporating an earth continuity conductor for connecting to the earthing contact or terminal of the appliance (except double insulated equipment).

A14   Lighting

Adequate and sufficient artificial or natural light for the task to be undertaken should be provided, with particular attention given to background and security lighting. This is particularly important at riding establishments where tuition may be undertaken in the evening and many visitors may not have knowledge of the topography of the area. Lights should be suitably protected or positioned so as not to present a hazard.

A15   Leading a horse on the highway

A15.1   Movement of horses across or along the public highway should always be undertaken in a prescribed safe manner and riders should be supervised and trained to adhere to safety procedures for horses as specified in the Highway Code.

A15.2   Horses led either on foot or from another horse should be on the left-hand side of the road and led from the handler's left, placing the handler between the horse and the traffic.

A15.3   A bridle should be worn when leading a horse on the public highway, and whenever leading a saddled horse, the stirrups should be 'run up' and secured.

A16   Loading and unloading facilities

A16.1   Adequate facilities for the safe loading and unloading of horses should be provided. Loading ramps should be anti-slip and not so steep as to cause alarm, and all permanently constructed ramps and platforms provided with adequate safety fencing and any sharp projections protected.

A16.2 Vehicles should comply with the Transit of Animals (Road and Rail) Orders.

A16.3 Personnel should not stand immediately beneath an opening or closing ramp.

A17 Lungeing manège

Lungeing should be carried out in a defined fenced manège by experienced, suitably trained personnel. Only those authorized or undergoing instruction should be permitted within the area during lungeing.

A18 Handling in confined areas

If horses have to be moved through confined spaces or near obstructions which may pose a risk to the handler, they should always be led. Simple handling tasks may be undertaken in the horse's own stable with adequate assistance, but more involved tasks are to be undertaken only when the horse has been correctly and appropriately restrained.

A19 Paddocks

A19.1 Care should be taken to ensure that paddocks are securely fenced, adequately gated and free from unnecessary obstructions. A horse should always be taken through the gate, well into the field and turned to face the entrance prior to release. An access gate should be provided with horse-proof latches.

A19.2 Grazing paddocks should be of adequate size for the number of horses contained.

A19.3 A horse should never be ridden into a paddock wearing only a head collar.

A20 Dress

A20.1 Footwear should be to the highest standards practicable, with a good heel to prevent the foot slipping through the stirrup iron. Whenever undertaking non-riding activities such as feeding, grooming, etc., so far as is reasonably practicable, staff should wear approved safety footwear.

A20.2 The high number of injuries which have occurred make it particularly important that riders as well as handlers who may be exposed to head injuries wear suitable protective headgear, correctly adjusted and fitted and conforming to (or surpassing) BS 6473: 1984. BS 4472: 1988 gives equally suitable protection. Instructors and proprietors should instigate spot checks to ensure that such headgear is correctly worn and adjusted. Furthermore, those handlers who may be exposed to risks of head injuries should be required to wear suitable protective headgear as described above.

Cycle helmets conforming to BS 6863: 1989 are listed as approved headgear in the Horses (Protective Headgear for Young Riders) Regulations 1992.

The above Regulations make it mandatory for children under 14 to wear protective headgear when riding on the road.

A20.3 Protective hats should be replaced periodically according to use and manufacturers' recommendations and damaged or dropped hats not worn until checked for safe use by the manufacturer or other expert person.

A20.4 Riders' and handlers' personal clothing should be maintained in good condition and be suitable for the purpose of use. The wearing of jewellery, e.g. earrings, is to be discouraged.

A21 Tack

A21.1 Rider safety and control of the horse may be seriously impaired unless all saddlery is in good condition and checked before use to ensure that it is safe and free from defects. Leather should be cleaned and regularly treated with particular care taken to identify damaged stitching. It is important that the tack provided for the horse on which the rider is to be mounted is suitable not only for the horse or pony but also for the particular rider, having regard to the rider's size, general riding ability and any known handicap or limitation.

A21.2 The saddle, if properly cared for, should last many years. However, certain parts need regular servicing and occasional replacement. Girth straps are stitched onto the webs which go over the tree (they should not be tacked on); this stitching will need to be redone occasionally and the straps may become worn and need replacing.

The stirrup leathers need their stitching checked regularly and their leather inspected for cracks or excess wear; replacement may save an accident. The safety catch on the stirrup bar of the saddle should be kept open when riding. Stirrups should be of stainless steel, or other high quality material, and must be of an appropriate size for the rider's feet. Bucket stirrups are useful for trekking and casual rider centres to cope with riders with inappropriate (cleated or soleless) footwear.

The bridle stitching should be inspected regularly. Buckles with bent tongues or loose hook studs should be replaced. Rein stops must be fitted with running martingales. Bits should be of good quality.

A21.3 Horse handling equipment and riding tack should be provided in sufficient quantity in relation to the type and number of horses housed at the establishment and adequate facilities should be available for restraining the horses when necessary.

A22   Staff training

A22.1   Under the Health and Safety at Work etc. Act 1974, employees must be given adequate instruction, training and supervision.

A22.2   Those who operate horse establishments should adopt a planned approach to training and supervision. Any instruction should include legal requirements, individual responsibilities, emergency procedures, e.g. in the event of fire or accident, reporting and monitoring arrangements, use of machinery, etc. Information on individual animals, machinery and substances should be passed on to employees together with correct safety procedures, and where there is a risk to health from livestock-transmissible disease, employees should be informed of the correct preventative measures. A copy of any written safety policy should be made available to all members of staff and explained fully.

A22.3   Training should consist of instruction and practice and include a development of the attitude, knowledge, skill and behaviour pattern required by an individual in order to perform safely a given task. Staff training should concentrate on safe systems of work. It should be made clear that safety and care in doing a job are more important than the speed at which it is carried out. No persons should be required to work with horses or other equipment unless they have received the necessary training for the work activity with refresher training provided when necessary.

A22.4   Supervision of employees is essential but its degree will depend on the level of training received. It is the responsibility of the employer to ensure that adequate training and supervision is provided for all employees with special emphasis placed on the less experienced. Any new employee should be closely supervised until the employer is satisfied that he or she is competent to undertake the duties required when a lesser degree of control will be sufficient. Non-employees who may be involved in the establishment's activities should receive similar supervision.

A23   Veterinary treatment

A23.1   It is recommended that veterinarians or farriers are assisted only by fully trained and experienced persons. Simple treatment may normally be undertaken within the horse's own stable. Complex treatment should only be administered if the horse is suitably and correctly restrained.

A23.2   Control is essential in the use of drugs and medicines due to the likelihood of injury by sharp instruments, e.g. hypodermic needles, and the fact that some products can be fatal to humans in the dose it would be necessary to administer to a horse.

A23.3   Drugs, medicines and treatments should only be held or administered by competent, nominated and fully trained personnel. Only these persons and those under their close supervision should have access to such products and manufacturers' and veterinary surgeons' instructions should be closely followed.

A23.4   All drugs, etc. should be separately and securely stored so that they are not accessible to unauthorized persons and a safe system of disposal of unwanted drugs, hypodermic syringes, etc. maintained.

A23.5   Veterinarians may use their own portable X-ray equipment at horse training establishments. The operator of this equipment will be responsible for ensuring its safe use but employers should be aware of the dangers and ensure that only nominated staff who have been fully instructed and protected are permitted to assist in radiography work. The Ionising Radiations Regulations 1985 apply to the use of this type of equipment.

A24   General housekeeping

A24.1   Many accidents result from trips and falls which may be prevented by good housekeeping. For example, hand tools, wheelbarrows, etc. should be correctly stored and hosepipes coiled onto reels and secured to a wall. Floors and stairways should be sound and well maintained to reduce the risk of injury.

A24.2   Accidents can be avoided if the means of access to the riding areas and any passages, paths or roads and any part of the premises to which employees or visitors have access, are kept clear of obstructions and have surfaces which minimize the risk of slipping.

A24.3   Pot-holes, broken steps, stairs or treads, uneven paving, holes in stable floors, defective gates and door fastenings, broken gates and doors, projections of wood or metal in unexpected places, passages blocked by barrels, buckets, bales of hay or straw, and forks or shovels lying about in or by any access ways are all potential hazards to visitors and employees at the premises. The proprietor should ensure that such hazards are not allowed to exist.

A25   Children

Care is necessary to ensure that children are not put at risk from work activities. Horses, machinery, buildings and chemicals can present particular risks to children and young people unless adequate precautions are taken. Additionally, fire, falls and falling objects, as well as drowning in grain slurry and water, have continued to cause unnecessary death or injury. The Agriculture (Avoidance of Accidents to Children) Regulations 1958 prohibit children under the age of 13 years from riding on or driving certain classes of vehicles or machines.

A26   Further information

Further information and advice on this subject may be obtained from the Health and Safety Executive.

PART B – ADDITIONAL SPECIFIC GUIDANCE FOR HORSE RIDING ESTABLISHMENTS

B1   Visitors

Riding establishments attract many persons with a limited knowledge of horses, and it is essential that instructors bring to their attention the dangers and procedures to be adopted to minimize the risk of injury. Arrangements should also be made to ensure that visitors are not exposed to danger and are, where appropriate, kept away from riding areas. If possible, a viewing area should be set aside and a clearly defined car parking area situated away from any collecting or training areas.

B2   Collecting yard

Most riding establishments provide a collecting area outside the stable blocks where riders mount, dismount or prepare for a riding lesson. Such areas should be level, well drained with adequate foot-hold and kept clean and free from obstruction except for devices provided for the safe mounting and dismounting of horses. Access and egress points should be suitably gated so that in an emergency horses are held within the confines of the collecting yard.

B3   Indoor schools

Ground surfaces should be so constructed as to afford adequate foot-hold. Doors should be of a sliding type or open outwards and be provided with kicking boards. Doors may open inwards providing the riding area is not obstructed. All doorways should be wide enough for the purpose of use. A suitable notice warning that entry should be made quietly and only after permission has been obtained should be permanently displayed. The perimeter of the school should be provided with a kicking board to a height of at least 1.35 m (4 ft 6 in) sloping outwards at an angle of 10° to 11°. Any obstructions or protrusions should be suitably protected by rollers or other effective means. Only an instructor, or a person authorized by the instructor, should be permitted within the school and all unnecessary equipment should be removed. Where necessary suitable arrangements should be made for spectators, perhaps by the provision of a viewing platform, with access to any spectators' area separated from that used by horse and rider.

Safe procedures for horses and people entering or leaving the school should be enforced.

B4   Riding paddocks and manèges

B4.1   If a paddock is used as an outdoor manège it should be of adequate size with a clear surface area free from obstructions or distractions which could upset the horse and rider, e.g. rabbit holes, electricity and telephone poles.

B4.2   All fencing should ideally be 1.5 m (5 ft) high but not less than 1.2 m (4 ft) and be secure and suitable for the purpose, e.g. post and rail with the rails facing inwards. Double fencing may also be used. Gates should be correctly hung to ensure that they open and close easily and have secure fastenings. Gates and side rails should be to a height of at least 1.5 m (5 ft) and gateways adequately maintained, e.g. free from mud.

B4.3   Manège size should correspond with normal dressage size arena, i.e. 20 m × 60 m or 20 m × 40 m, or reduced proportionately where space dictates that a horse can be worked/exercised in a reasonable shape and riders are in a more easily controlled situation/environment. Jumps or similar hazards should be constructed where possible on level ground unless the standard of instruction requires otherwise. Take-off and landing areas should always be maintained in good condition, inspected prior to use and, if riders are not undertaking instruction in jumping technique, equipment dismantled and moved to a safe area.

B5   Rider selection

B5.1   Only persons with adequate experience should be allowed to ride a horse which is known to be excitable, or to ride at a gallop. It is essential that acts of bravado are immediately suppressed and especially when both males and females ride out together. If horses unavoidably have been boxed for several days prior to riding out, they should first be lunged or exercised and extra care taken to ensure that only experienced riders have charge of the animals.

B5.2   Instructors should ensure that the horse or pony provided for a rider's use is suitable and safe in the particular circumstances, taking into account age, size, experience, general riding ability and any known handicap or limitation of the rider.

B5.3   The instructor should also ensure that students are not asked or given permission to do any act of horse management or riding unless it is believed to be within their capabilities.

B6   Selection of instructors

B6.1   No person under the age of 16 should be left in control of an establishment, be permitted to instruct or be in control of a lesson.

B6.2   It is essential that any person put in charge of a ride or lesson is properly qualified and is sufficiently responsible to be left in such a position. Instructors should have experience for the task they are required to undertake, be competent handlers of horses and, preferably, hold appropriate qualifications.

B6.3   The BHS maintains a Register of Instructors who are held to be competent by way of qualifications, who hold insurance and who regularly attend training courses. They are also required to have training in first-aid.

B7   Instructor/student ratios

B7.1   Although circumstances may permit certain variations, it is recommended that the following instructor/student ratios are adhered to during riding:
(1)   Assistant instructor: 4 students.
(2)   Intermediate instructor: 5–8 students.
(3)   Instructor: 7–10 students.

B7.2   In addition, it is recommended that for hacks no more than six riders be under the care of one instructor, who should be at least 16 years of age and competent to supervise a hack. This does not preclude clients going on an individual hack if the proprietor is satisfied that the client is competent to ride without supervision.

B7.3   Any significant variation from these ratios may only be made following consideration by a responsible person who is competent to make a decision based on experience and knowledge of the instructor, riders and horses, and the type of lesson being undertaken.

B8 Group rides

B8.1 The group should not be asked or allowed to do anything which will endanger the weakest rider who may lack ability or experience. The ride should be kept under close supervision by an experienced person and so conducted that no horse is left behind or likely to lose sight of the remainder of the ride.

B8.2 Group rides should be organized so that:
- (1) the least experienced riders are on the quietest horses;
- (2) riders with least experience are in the middle of the ride;
- (3) young or nervous horses are positioned on the inside of an older experienced horse but under no circumstances should riders ride more than two abreast; and
- (4) experienced riders are always at the front and rear of the ride.

B9 Staff training

B9.1 Under the Health and Safety at Work etc. Act 1974 employees must be given adequate instruction, training and supervision, the detail and extent of which will vary depending on the staff concerned who may be:
- (1) qualified instructors or persons of equivalent experience;
- (2) students under training to attain qualifications as instructors; or
- (3) regular employees with or without horse experience.

B9.2 The training of employees should take into account that there will be other people at the school including:
- (1) volunteer workers, i.e. those who carry out horse handling tasks to gain experience and/or in exchange for riding out;
- (2) paying clients who are receiving a recognized course of instruction; and
- (3) clients whose horses are kept on a livery basis.

B9.3 Instructional staff should have experience or qualifications appropriate to the standard to which they are instructing. Qualifications will include a certificate(s) received as a result of formal training.

B10 Horse care

B10.1 It is essential to ensure that adequate and qualified assistance is available for any treatment administered to the horse. In particular, horse clipping should only be undertaken by a fully trained person assisted by an experienced horse handler.

B10.2 Students and clients should only be permitted to groom animals, pick hooves, etc. when the instructor is satisfied that they are competent to undertake such tasks. Care needs to be taken to ensure that no visitors are permitted within the area where such operations are taking place in case of distraction to either horse or student.

B11   Tack fitting and care

Instructors or other persons with sufficient knowledge should always ensure that tack is correctly fitted, in good condition and suitable for the horse or pony before a rider receives any instruction.

PART C – ADDITIONAL SPECIFIC GUIDANCE FOR STUDS AND HORSE BREEDING ESTABLISHMENTS

C1   Covering yard

This is usually an enclosed area for both weather protection and ease of horse handling. The enclosed building should be approximately 18.25 m × 10.5 m (60 ft × 35 ft) and provided with adequate natural and artificial lighting. The floor area should be level, free from dust and obstruction and afford adequate foot-hold for both handler and horse. Generally two doorways should be provided at opposite ends, one for the stallion and one for the mare. Single doors should be a minimum of 1.35 m (4 ft 6 in) wide and it is recommended that side rollers are fitted. Ideally, one set should be double doors to permit easy access to the building for the removal of fouled bedding. Internal walls should be free from projections, with corners and stanchions rounded or protected by rollers.

C2   Trying board or gate

This facility can either be incorporated as part of the covering yard or built outside in the open as a permanent structure. It should be robustly constructed of heavy timber with sufficient padding on either side and a rolling bar of at least 100 mm (4 in) diameter along the top. All sharp edges should be bevelled or rounded and the trying bar of sufficient height to permit the stallion to get only his head and neck over.

C3   Trying the mare

It is recommended that the stallion is held back from the bar until the mare is in a suitable position. In confined areas a recess should be provided near the mare's head to allow the handler to step back out of the risk area should the mare rear up and strike out.

C4 Horse covering

During covering at least three experienced persons should be present comprising the recognized stallion handler and two other fully trained horse handlers. The stallion handler should be in control of the stallion and the covering procedure, with another person in control of the mare to be covered and the remaining person in attendance at the rear of the mare. The mare throughout the covering period should be wearing covering boots on her hind feet.

C5 Foaling boxes

Foaling boxes should be as large as possible and at least 4.25 m × 4.5 m (14 ft × 15 ft). Adequate artificial and natural lighting should be provided. It is recommended that there should be no fixtures or fittings within the box other than a manger and water point with the areas underneath infilled. Doors should be constructed to open outwards in two halves, fitted with anti-slide bolts and provided with a kick latch at the base of the lower door. Floors should be free from obstruction, anti-slip and, in the interests of hygiene, impervious, easily cleansed and disinfected.

C6 Sitting-up room

C6.1 If a sitting-up room is provided, there should be access to the foaling box and a window provided for observation into the box. Closed-circuit TV cameras should be so positioned that they create no risk to either horse or person. Adequate welfare facilities should be provided, e.g. suitable furniture, heating, washing and toilet facilities. Drugs, medicines and disinfectants should be kept in a secure, locked cupboard nearby and not within the room. Provision should also be made for the storage of extra tack, head collars, ropes, etc.

C6.2 Sitting-up rooms should be provided with a telephone or other facility to enable regular contact to be maintained with a lone person. Whenever someone is required to sit-up, a system of regular contact should be established to ensure that he or she is not unsupervised for long periods. No attempt should be made by a lone person to attend the mare unless assistance has been summoned.

C7 Age

The age, experience and physique of personnel should be taken into account when deciding if they should handle stallions. In general, handlers should be over 18 and under 65 years old. Younger persons are unlikely to have the necessary mental or physical capabilities or be sufficiently experienced to handle a stallion.

In no circumstances should they be allowed to do so unless under the supervision of an older person who has received the necessary training in the handling of such animals.

C8 Visitors

Breeding establishments can and do attract many authorized visitors such as owners, contractors, delivery persons, etc. In such situations, arrangements should be made to ensure that visitors are aware of the dangers of horses and are, as far as possible, kept away from areas of risk. It is recommended that all visitors are confined, in the first instance, to a reception area until accompanied by an experienced and authorized person having a working knowledge of the establishment.

C9 Leading in and out of paddocks

Breeding establishments adopt many methods of leading in and out and it is essential that a safe procedure for this operation is devised to minimize the risk of injury to both horse and handler especially if several animals are involved at one time.

PART D – ADDITIONAL SPECIFIC GUIDANCE FOR RACEHORSE TRAINING ESTABLISHMENTS

D1 General public

Training gallops can be situated on land to which the general public may have access. In such situations, arrangements should be made to ensure that the public are aware of the dangers of horses and are, so far as possible, kept away from the area. If training areas adjoin a public highway, consideration should be given to the provision of suitable fencing to contain a recalcitrant horse. Attention needs to be drawn to the importance of keeping pets under proper control and it is recommended that they are prohibited from such areas during training periods. It is also recommended that all visitors to stables are confined, in the first instance, to a reception area until accompanied by an experienced and authorized person having a working knowledge of the establishment.

D2 Training gallops

The majority of injuries are sustained while exercising horses. Falls on the gallops occur for a variety of reasons, e.g. high spirited animals, horses stumbling and lack of adequate training, instruction and supervision of riders. It is essential that whilst exercising horses, riders are properly supervised and make correct use of the appropriate equipment. Young or excitable horses are less likely to become unsettled if they are taken to the gallops in strings rather than singly, and this method should be used wherever possible. The training gallops must be well maintained and free from obstructions to reduce the risk of injury to horse or rider whilst travelling at speed. Young persons of below school leaving age should not be allowed to participate in riding out.

D3   Training aids

The correct training of horses for racecourse procedures is seen to be an essential factor in the reduction of racing accidents. Trainers with a flat licence should have access to practice starting stalls to familiarize both horses and staff with the equipment. Similarly, schooling practice fences should be available for steeple chasers and hurdlers. No horse should be entered for any race unless appropriately trained or schooled.

D4   Covered exercise area

Ground surfaces should be so constructed and maintained as to afford adequate foot-hold. The ride-way should be of sufficient width with kick boards at least 1.35 m (4 ft 6 in) high, away from the track preferably at an angle of 10° to 11°. Pedestrians should not be permitted access to the exercise track while horses are present, except in an emergency. A viewing box or platform is desirable and riders should be adequately supervised.

D5   Rider selection

Only riders with adequate experience should be allowed to ride a horse which is known to be excitable or to ride at a gallop. It is essential to ensure, particularly when young staff ride out together, that acts of bravado are immediately suppressed. If horses have been boxed for several days prior to riding out, extra care needs to be taken to ensure that only experienced riders have charge of the animals.

D6   Staff training

Under the Health and Safety at Work etc. Act 1974, employees must be given adequate instruction, training and supervision. Although racehorse trainers are expected to give 'on the job' theoretical and practical training, more formal training may also be required, e.g. in the case of young or inexperienced employees. The British Racing School, Newmarket, for example, organizes Basic Courses for stable lads and stable girls as well as Advanced Courses for apprentice jockeys.

Appendix 2: National Vocational Qualifications

Introduction to Vocational Qualifications (S/NVQs)

National Vocational Qualifications are designed to accredit skills. The basis for their development was threefold. Firstly, the British Government wanted a national scheme, with uniformity between industries, which clarified skill recognition throughout the country and overseas. Secondly, formal examinations are not always the best way of assessing achievement in a vocational area. It is logical that a person's ability to do a craft-based job should be judged by seeing how capable they are at doing every task and working under a variety of circumstances. Thirdly, it is recognized that in many walks of life people learn their craft by experience and this is the basis of good workmanship; so it is good to have a system for accrediting those skills which allows ongoing progress to be monitored and which is sufficiently flexible to cope with individuals' situations.

National Vocational Qualifications (NVQs) are a useful system for recognizing and encouraging achievement which, when properly used, can offer benefits to all areas of the horse industry. In Scotland there is a similar system, so to cover both, these vocational qualifications may be referred to as S/NVQs. In some areas these systems run in parallel with other, older examination systems.

During the development of S/NVQs the horse industry was constrained by the National Council for Vocational Qualifications; unfortunately that body proved both bureaucratic and dictatorial. It also made a number of mistakes, so in the late 1980s and early 1990s the proposed system was changed several times and this led to some confusion. Hopefully the National Council for VQs will now follow the advice given by the Joint National Horse Education and Training Council (JNHETC), on behalf of the horse industry, and aim for a decade of stability and coherence, so that the system can settle down and be more clearly understood.

NVQs are based on levels of competence with Level 1 being the first achieved and higher levels progressively calling for more skill and knowledge. For each NVQ level there follows a description of the person's capabilities, a title that could be used to describe their job and an outline of their skills. The skills listed below refer to horsemanship in any sector of the industry, but the levels also cater for specialist skills such as riding, driving, stud work, racing, heavy horses and so on.

NVQ Level 1

A person working at Level 1 may lack depth of experience of horse work or, for some reason, have limited skills. He or she is capable of simple routine tasks in and around the stable yard but requires a good deal of supervision and should only work with reasonably quiet horses. The job title might be Trainee Groom, Assistant Groom or Stable Assistant.

The skills required are:

- *Horsemastership skills*
  Feeding and watering to a set ration and routine.
  Rugging up and unrugging.
  Cleaning tack and rugs.
  Receiving and storing hay, straw and feed.
  Keeping yards in tidy condition.
  Turning horses out, recognizing them and catching them.
  Routine tacking up and untacking.
  Grooming and washing horses.
- *Receiving and assisting visitors to the yard*
- *Liaising with visitors and colleagues*
- *Operating safely in the workplace.*

Most importantly of all, a Level 1 employee needs to be co-operative with workmates, polite to visitors and should understand why things are being done and the dangers of failing to follow good practice.

NVQ Level 2

This person is competent at routine tasks. He or she is able to work efficiently and, in the normal course of events, needs only minimal supervision. The Level 2 employee is observant and has the confidence to tell the Head Girl or Head Lad about any problems or changes to the norm which may need ongoing observations. Horse terminology is understood and this employee can therefore carry out more complicated instructions. Although only able to cope with horses behaving in a calm manner, this person can act as a useful assistant to a more senior member of staff dealing with a fractious horse or more difficult situation. The job title might be Groom, or in racing, Lad.

The skills required are:

- *Horsemastership skills*
  Watering and feeding – to an agreed ration.
  Bandaging (stable and travel bandages).
  Cleaning and storing rugs.
  Pulling and plaiting a mane.
  Grooming and checking shoes.

Tacking up and untacking for performance, exercise or lungeing.
Presenting horse for inspection for soundness.
Assessing horse for health and recognizing lameness.
Caring for a sick horse as instructed.
Basic handling.
Lungeing a quiet horse as instructed.
Caring for a horse at grass including checking fields.
Assisting with horse transportation.
- *Develop and maintain personal effectiveness*
  Be a good communicator.
  Have self discipline and good working practices.
- *Optional skill areas*
  Riding horses.
  Working with racehorses.
  Working with breeding stock.
  Assisting with working and driving horses.

In terms of attitude to work, Level 2 employees should give consideration to ways in which they can make their own work better and more efficient; they should work thoughtfully, positively and cheerfully. They need some understanding of how people work together in teams and need to be co-operative and responsible.

NVQ Level 3

The Level 3 worker has gained considerable experience. He or she is capable of dealing with most situations and uses initiative. This employee has the self-discipline to work alone and in a team. Often someone at this level will be responsible for the training and supervision of junior staff and so will be able to show a thorough knowledge of horsemastership and personnel skills. The usual job title is Head Girl or Yard Manager. In racing, the Head Lad of a large yard will be a person with Level 4 experience and will take responsibility and remuneration to match.

The skills required at Level 3 are:

- *Horsemastership skills*
  Provide routine health care (feet, vaccinations, worming, etc.).
  Identify unsoundness, injury or ill-health.
  Treat health problems as advised by vet or manager.
  Compile feed chart and order feed in consultation with the manager.
  Travelling horses.
- *Supervisory skills*
  Contribute to the training and development of teams, individuals and self to enhance performance.

Contribute to the planning, organization and evaluation of work.
Create, maintain and enhance productive working relationships.
>   NB These three units are explained and discussed in greater detail later in
>   this section.

- *Optional skill areas*
  Preparing horses for work including clipping.
  Riding horses to maintain particular training.
  Working draught or driving horses.
  Driving horses on the road.
  Working and schooling racehorses.
  Taking horses racing.
  Stud work.
  Rearing young horses.
- *Additional skill areas*
  Grassland care.
  Trekking.
  Estate care.
  Assisting disabled riders.
  Coaching the rider.

The Level 3 employee needs to have a thorough understanding of the nature of the business and of how the various aspects fit together to achieve the optimum result. This person often has a wide span of control and may represent the business to clients and visitors. He or she will set an example of good attitude and good practice.

NVQ Level 4

In comparative terms, the practical horse industry consists mostly of small businesses in which the person at Level 4 is the manager and possibly also the owner. This role consists principally of arranging the strategy of the business. The most important considerations in ensuring the long-term success of an enterprise include monitoring present performance and assessing alternative business plans which use the resources of the yard to best advantage. The span of control is very wide and touches on all aspects of the business. This person should lead from the front and set an appropriate style and enthusiasm. The usual title is Manager.

The skills required are:

Maintain and improve the condition of horses.
Create, manage and maintain a suitable environment – yard facilities.
Manage the operation – activities, finance, people and information.
Market the operation.
>   NB These last three are the principal subject matter of this book.

- *Optional skill areas*
  Breeding – policy and supervising or organizing key activities.
  Rearing – policy and key activities.
  Select, break and train horses to optimize their potential.
  Race riding.
  Competition riding.
  Teaching and coaching.

NVQ structure within each level

It can be seen that the framework of NVQs fits closely with the general nature of progression within the horse industry. An important quality of NVQs is the flexibility they offer. To understand how this works in practice consider the structure of an NVQ level.

NVQs are broken down into units which each represent an area of skill. For each level there are mandatory units and optional units. NVQs are assembled like building blocks. The complete NVQ at any level indicates that a person has the essential skills to work at that level.

NVQ = mandatory units + optional units

Mandatory units plus at least one optional unit have to be completed by anyone who wants to achieve the NVQ qualification. The mandatory units comprise knowledge or skill that is essential across all areas of the horse industry.

Optional units comprise the essential skills for a particular area of the industry. They enable people to tailor the NVQs to their own experience. So a person working in a racing yard can do the mandatory units concerning care of the horse plus optional units in use of the racehorse. Another person may be making a career in horse breeding. This person would complete the same mandatory units but would add an optional unit in stud work.

The flexibility of NVQs rests primarily on individuals being able to choose units in an area and at a level that suits their current experience.

As well as the units needed to gain a level, a person may take other optional units or additional units to show their extra breadth of knowledge and skill; they may also take higher level units to show their extra skill in certain areas.

NVQ methods of assessment

NVQs check that work is consistent by requiring that evidence of good work is collected over a period of time. The person responsible for judging that evidence is an Assessor who has been trained in judging competence. Any experienced person can train to become an Assessor so it may be that a worker who wants to gain an NVQ qualification could be assessed by their own supervisor. At first this might seem to be open to abuse but in reality it is not, for two reasons: firstly, whenever an Assessor signs to say that a person is up to standard they are putting their own professional reputation on the line; secondly, the work of the Assessor is checked by a Verifier. If the Assessor's work is not up to standard they must either retrain or stop being an Assessor.

Most people working with horses operate at a variety of levels; it is possible to have a 'Level 1 hat on' for morning yards and a 'Level 3 hat on' for training staff – and perhaps a 'Level 4 hat on' to arrange a bank loan!

The skills of horsemastership required for NVQ Levels 1, 2 and 3 are fully discussed in J. Houghton Brown and S. Pilliner's book *Horse Care* and J. Houghton Brown and V. Powell-Smith's book *Horse and Stable Management* Second edition. The skills of management at NVQ Level 4 are the subject of other sections of this book.

The remainder of this section is devoted to a discussion of the requirements of NVQ Level 3 managerial and supervisory skills.

NVQ Level 3 – Management and supervisory units

In their current form the management and supervisory units at NVQ Level 3 are at first sight difficult to understand; they are written in the complex language of management training. The aim of this section is to demystify the requirements of achieving these units. It is hoped that the NVQ requirements themselves will be more clearly stated in future, but this is subject to the National Council for Vocational Qualifications. The Joint National Horse Education and Training Council, on behalf of the horse industry, has always sought to use simple, easily understood, plain English appropriate to the work under consideration.

The competent supervisor, using Level 3 skills, acts between the manager of the business, who may be the owner, and the other people who work there. The supervisory skills required for NVQ Level 3 are summarized below:

- *Organizational*
  Planning work to be done.
  Ensuring that it is done on time to agreed procedures.
  Assessing the quality of work done.
  Telling people whether work is good enough or not and if not, why.
  Adjusting the planning and organization of work for greater efficiency.
- *Training*
  Understanding the strengths and weaknesses of staff, i.e. what they are and are not good at.
  Defining training needs to ensure that staff are able to do the work that they are asked to do.
  Planning training to improve staff skills.
  Delivering training to improve staff skills.
  Checking progress and learning from the training.

- *Personnel*
  Creating a united team which works coherently.
  Ensuring individuals work harmoniously.
  Passing information from management to staff and from staff to management.
  Motivating staff and applying disciplinary procedures.

It is impossible to separate totally the various threads of supervisory skills. They are like a rope; the strength of the rope (or of the business) depends not only on the strength of the individual strands but also on the way they are twisted together.

Level 3 – Organization skills

Planning and organizing work

A competent person working at Level 3 is responsible for the day-to-day planning and organization of work. The importance of this area of responsibility cannot be over-estimated. It is fundamental to achieving the aims of the business.

The first consideration of planning work is what has to be achieved today, this week and this month. A good way of planning work is to look at the diary for the coming week. Typical things to be completed may include: a farrier's visit to trim all youngstock's feet; a large delivery of hay arriving; and some fields to be topped and harrowed because stock has just been moved into fresh grazing.

All these tasks need the right people to do the job; they may need some preparation so that the actual work goes smoothly and the people concerned need some warning so that they can work efficiently.

To organize such work it is useful to have short daily and weekly staff meetings. These provide an opportunity to inform staff of what is proposed and to make arrangements to ensure that the work goes smoothly. Such work planning meetings ensure that staff understand the whole picture.

Using the example given above, typical problems and solutions that may be raised at such a weekly staff meeting are as follows:

Farrier's visit

There are twelve youngstock to have their feet trimmed. The farrier will need two people to catch and hold the horses. Anne has got a BHS Stage II exam shortly and would benefit from watching and talking to the farrier. John is good at handling unruly youngstock and will enable the process to go smoothly. John and Anne will be occupied half of the day and so their ordinary work needs to be given to other members of staff.

Hay delivery

The driver plus three people are needed to unload, but not Jane because she has asthma. Clare, the new trainee, is working for NVQ Level 1 and so needs to be experienced at handling bales. The barn needs clearing of old hay, the floor swept and pallets putting down. This can be done over a series of days whenever five minutes are available.

The old hay is very dusty and dust masks will be needed.

Paddocks

This is not very urgent, but needs to be done when the ground is dry and preferably on the horse's rest day so that the routine workload is lighter. The tractor will be working hard with the mower and so needs oil and water checking and the power-take-off (PTO) greasing. The PTO cover is cracked and needs replacing before it is used again so this component needs ordering at once.

Even in these simple examples, many aspects of work are considered; there is a productive exchange of information. The right people are given jobs according to their talents and training needs; many potential problems are foreseen and adherence to health and safety legislation is demonstrated.

It is not enough to plan work and hope that all goes well; it is also necessary to monitor the work as it goes on. This does not mean that a supervisor should need to watch over somebody's shoulder. For example, when the hay is almost unloaded and working space is cramped it may be better for the supervisor to suggest that one person starts raking up any spilled hay or broken bales.

The most important aspect of monitoring and evaluating work done is to ask for feedback from the people doing the work. If the Head Girl was to ask Clare (the trainee) how she got on she may be given the following information:

- The work rate was too fast to begin with.
- The pattern of stacking bales was not explained.
- It was difficult to lift properly and keep up the speed.

The next time the Head Girl briefs staff on unloading hay she may make the following points:

- Work as a team – only go as fast as everyone can manage.
- More experienced members of a team need to explain to novices as they go so that everyone understands the job in hand.
- Safe practice must not be forgotten because of eagerness to get the job done.

The process of planning, monitoring and evaluating work need not take up a lot of time. The benefits, in constantly improving the way jobs are done, very quickly improve the efficiency of the business.

Level 3 – Training Skills

Planning, delivering and evaluating training

In most yards it is impossible to separate training from ordinary work. The new recruit learns from the explanations of yard practice, for example *why* horses are tied up to be mucked out. The more competent person learns from striving to do a better job and from asking questions.

Part of the ethos of NVQs is that people at all levels should be personally responsible for setting their own goals for improvement. However, this needs encouragement, guidance and the provision of more formal training as necessary. It is recognized that training is an investment in the staff and in the business, but it can be expensive in money and time, so needs to be well planned.

One starting point in planning training is the agreed progression of individual staff members based on their contracts and annual appraisal review meetings. Another starting point is an analysis of the needs of the business. This is then compared with the skills that staff have already and where the two do not match there is a need for training. Once again it is worthwhile planning ahead so that skills are in place when they are needed. It may be that the owner of a business wants to expand the teaching of private clients. This requires that staff who have not previously done much teaching will find themselves doing more. It is to everyone's benefit that teaching skills are improved before the clients arrive. The teaching staff are happier because they are more confident in teaching, the clients are happier because they have better lessons and the owner is happier because those clients are satisfied and come back for more lessons.

Having established what training needs exist within the business, the question of who should be trained arises. There is little point in training somebody for an area of work they are not keen to improve. Acquiring or improving skills is a partnership process requiring effort from the trainee as well as the trainer.

Once the training needs have been identified and the trainee sees the benefits of training, a decision has to be made on the best way of training. The two most common routes are to use in-house skills so a senior staff member may train a junior, or to use external resources by sending a person on a course or to a conference. The former method is less expensive but brings no new ideas into the business. So the most effective procedure is to use both methods and to ensure that all relevant staff benefit from an explanation when a delegate returns from external training. If training is carried out in-house the principles of learning explained in Chapter 3 must be applied.

The enormous cost of training dictates that it must be as effective as possible, so after any training session or programme a review should be made of how effective the training has been and whether alternative methods may be effective. This principle applies from simple schemes to grand schemes. For example, the senior instructor may recommend that juniors watch a video concerning the rider's position, but if the senior instructor is not available to answer any questions arising from the video, part of the potential value of training is lost. Similarly, paying for a junior instructor to go to a specialist convention may not provide value for money because the level is too high. It would be much better for the senior instructor to go and to pass on information at a level that the junior instructor can understand.

Providing information about training is also important. A properly scheduled programme of lectures, for instance, allows the trainee to collect his/her thoughts about the subject well beforehand. Formal or informal tests or observation of the trainee's work enable the trainer to monitor the progress and effectiveness of training and provide an opportunity for the trainer to reassure the trainee that improvement is being shown.

Self-improvement

When a large part of a person's work role involves supervising others and encouraging or training them to work well, it is easy to forget self-improvement. It is just as important for supervisors to strive constantly to improve as it is for junior employees.

A self checklist is given below which covers many similar points that a supervisor needs to assess when considering trainees.

- What skills do I have now?
- What skills need improving?
- What new skills may I need to serve the aims of the business?
- How am I going to meet those training needs?
- How will I tell if I am getting better?
- Who should I go to for an objective opinion of my progress?

Level 3 – Personnel skills

Good working relationships with colleagues and juniors

The supervisor is the focus for information from all sorts of people. Sometimes queries can be dealt with immediately or sometimes the supervisor will need to either pass on the problem to another person, perhaps to the owner of the business. Passing the right information to the right people in the right way is essential to the smooth running of a business.

The first priority for dealing with people is that the supervisor must be accessible. That is to say that if a new employee has a problem, they must feel that the supervisor is willing to listen and to try and sort the problem out.

Staff meetings are an ideal forum for staff to raise work-related problems, but the supervisor should be aware that it is not the right place to discuss employees' personal problems.

Offer advice helpfully

Often it takes some courage for an employee or other person to raise a problem. No matter how insignificant a problem may seem, the person raising it must feel that it has been taken seriously and must be satisfied with the action taken. Often the supervisor can deal with the matter there and then but he/she should also recognize when a solution is beyond his/her control and should be prepared to pass it on to a specialist.

Keep promises
The outcome of any discussion should be an action plan to improve the situation. It is very important that everyone does what they say they will do. Sometimes plans have to be amended and if so the supervisor needs to explain why.

Keep people informed
It is frustrating to feel that only 'lip service' has been given to a problem. Everybody needs to know the outcome of their problem or suggestion. Even if nothing can be done it is better to know that and to know the reason why nothing can be done.

The principles mentioned above are applied here to a practical problem.

- Problem: The Head Girl is concerned that morning yards are taking too long and that staff are tired because they are starting earlier in the morning to get the yards finished by 08.00.
- Consultation: The matter is raised at a staff meeting and ideas to improve things are sought.
- Suggestion: Fitting automatic water bowls would make yards quicker and easier for staff.
- Proposed action: Head Girl will discuss fitting water bowls with the yard owner.
- Discussion with owner: Water bowls are too expensive at present. Make new proposals.
- Amended plan: A trough and dip bucket will be placed near stables to speed up bucket-filling and minimize carrying.
- Explanation to staff: Water bowls are too expensive at the moment, but a dip tank is being arranged and this is how it is to be used. If this causes any problems let the Head Girl know.
- New working practice:

    (1) The trough is to be emptied and refilled weekly.
    (2) Only the dip-bucket is to be used for filling stable buckets and this must be put back on its hook after use – it must never be set down on the ground.
    (3) Care must be taken not to overfill buckets and spill water, especially in icy weather.

Good working relationships with own superior
In the example just given, the Head Girl had to refer to the owner about having automatic water bowls fitted. This section uses the same example to illustrate how the Head Girl can ensure good communication with the owner of the yard.

Firstly, the Head Girl needs to explain the problem with the right level of detail. In this case the personalities of staff and horses are irrelevant. The problem centres around the efficient provision of water.

The method of explanation is also important. In this case it would be good to get the yard owner to see how inefficient it is to carry buckets long distances. A written explanation would not be as effective.

Proposals for improvement need to be clearly stated. The principle here is providing automated drinkers. The particular type is not important at this stage.

When the yard owner does not accept the proposal for reasons of cost, the Head Girl must try to find alternative solutions. In this case, providing a dip tank was the affordable solution.

Management of conflict

Effective work depends on people working happily and efficiently together. Interpersonal conflict causes team spirit to fail or not to be achieved at all. The causes of conflict can be many and varied and the effective supervisor needs to be aware of them. Some examples of the causes of conflict are given below.

- Differences of opinion on method or standard of work.
- Personal animosity.
- Racial or sexual prejudice.
- Personal habits including smoking and housekeeping standards.
- Team roles.

The nature of work in the horse industry is such that people often work long hours under arduous conditions, and particularly where staff share accommodation the potential for conflict is high. It is because of the need to minimize conflict that a principal criterion for selecting staff is whether they will 'fit in' with the style of the business and the existing staff.

There is so much potential for conflict in the workplace that it is sensible to set policy on as many areas of performance as possible. For example, all employees must conform to the requirements of the organization. Such an agreement forms part of the employee's terms of employment. Items that should be mentioned in an employee's terms of employment may include standards of dress, wearing of jewellery and time-keeping. Where accommodation is provided, a policy regarding housekeeping standards and receiving visitors is essential.

Having clear written policies on as many areas of employment as possible reduces the room for misunderstanding and provides a clear point of reference should disciplinary procedures be necessary.

Much conflict in the horse world arises out of real or imagined unfair treatment or favouritism. The yard supervisor may have various strategies to avoid conflict. The first is to be aware of potential hazards and to minimize their effects. An example of such a situation might be a new employee who shares accommodation with two current employees. The three of them may well settle in and live happily together; or the new recruit could do less than a fair share of housework; or the two current residents may load the work onto the new person.

In this situation the potential conflict is reduced by asking the two current residents to devise a housework rota for a three-person household. Devising a rota ensures that the current residents are reminded of the need to allocate work fairly, and in the event of the new recruit not pulling his or her weight it serves as a starting point for a discussion among the three residents.

When actual conflict arises it is very important to act quickly. What may begin as a minor irritation soon develops into a festering sore. Employees must be encouraged to approach their supervisor and they will only do that if they feel the supervisor will be fair and treat the complaint confidentially.

It is very important and only fair to hear both sides of the story. Handling situations with a light touch is important. Perhaps a general chat about the importance of teamwork on the way to a show will be enough to prick the conscience of an employee who disappears when the muck heap needs tidying.

It is important also to recognize and reward improvement. Commenting on the admirable state of the muck heap when everyone has done the job together encourages repeatedly good work.

Of course not all conflicts can be dealt with so informally. When problems continue, a more formal approach is required which may eventually lead to a disciplinary procedure. For this reason, taking accurate notes of even small incidents is important.

Implementing disciplinary and grievance procedures

Specific details of disciplinary and grievance procedures are to be found in Chapters 3 and 5. These are always unpleasant situations to deal with, but having a set procedure that ensures all the appropriate stages of investigation and warnings have been followed ensures that the process is fair to all concerned and can be concluded at an early stage.

Criteria for a good equestrian worker

A good equestrian worker:

- Takes responsibility to do each job, however simple, to the best of his/her ability. Takes pride and interest in his/her work.
- Is reliable. The job will be done as and when agreed and if this proves impossible the good equestrian worker will communicate that fact at the earliest opportunity.
- Uses time efficiently. This is partly a matter of thinking fast and partly a matter of being well prepared. It is also essential to be punctual.
- Brings to the work a range of skills based on sound training, experience and a good attitude to horses.
- Knows his/her own limitations yet is keen to extend knowledge and skills.

- Uses initiative and yet is willing to say when he/she does not understand or does not know how to do a task or needs assistance.
- Takes a responsible attitude to safety. Obeys the safety code. Adheres to established (good, safe) practice. Never puts others at risk.
- Understands the principles and practice of animal welfare in the context of the performance of horses.
- Is loyal and a good ambassador with a pleasant manner and a tidy appearance.

Criteria for a good team member

A good team member:

- Appreciates corporate responsibility. Jobs must all be completed to a high standard. It is up to *everyone* to see that this happens.
- Makes an effort to establish and maintain good relationships with other members of the team. (Sometimes other team members can be difficult; sometimes one feels in a bad mood; so it is important to 'make an effort'.) Getting on with others should not be taken for granted.
- Makes an effort to establish and maintain a good relationship with his/her supervisor (Head Girl, etc.) or employer. Sometimes they may seem grumpy but maybe they are preoccupied with other problems.
- Meets strangers or visitors to the yard positively, politely and helpfully. There has to be an agreed procedure for dealing with visitors for their own safety, for yard efficiency and for security.
- Communicates well. Good relationships and good team achievement are aided by letting others know what is happening.
- Listens, remembers or records and passes on messages accurately and speedily.

Criteria for a good supervisor

A good supervisor:

- Selects safe, efficient and effective ways of doing all routine tasks, and insists that staff (including trainees, etc.) do tasks the proper way.
- Appreciates that a good relationship with the team is a two-way process and shows authority and sensitivity in making it work.
- Listens, discusses, justifies and yet is always willing to accept improvements.
- Advises, demonstrates, refers and helps to achieve individual and team high performance.
- Deals with problems clearly and pleasantly, including problems concerned with jobs or with colleagues.

- Is reliable, both from the viewpoint of the employer and the other team members. A good supervisor will always do his/her best, both for the employer and for the staff and, where their respective needs conflict, the supervisor has to enforce the employer's requirements with tact, loyalty and authority. It is sometimes a tough job!
- Is a good communicator.
- Can bring in change with understanding, clarity and continuity.
- Can use authority without giving rise to resentment.
- Can maintain standards of quality, tidiness and, where appropriate, work output.
- Can counsel colleagues by listening and helping them to reflect wisely on possible alternative solutions, encouraging colleagues towards self-help.

Index